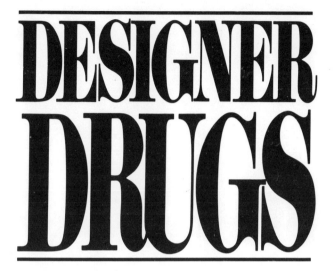

M.M. KIRSCH

CompCare Publications
2415 Annapolis Lane
Minneapolis, Minnesota 55441

Kirsch, M.M., 1954–
    Designer drugs.

    Bibliography: p. 169
    Includes index.
    1. Designer drugs.   2. Drug abuse—United States.
I. Title.
RM316.K57   1986   362.2'93   86-23249
ISBN 0-89638-109-9

Cover design by David Hada
Cover consultation, interior design by Susan Rinek
Index by Audrey E. DeLaMartre

Inquiries, orders, and catalog requests should be addressed to
CompCare Publications
2415 Annapolis Lane
Minneapolis, Minnesota 55441
Call toll free 800/328-3330
(Minnesota residents 559-4800)

9   8   7   6   5   4   3   2   1

90   89   88   87   86

Special thanks to Oliver Horeczky

Contents

Tell me, I'll forget. Show me, I may remember.
But involve me, and I'll understand.

Chinese Proverb

Introduction

Designer drugs are subverting the black-market drug trade, undermining and diverting law enforcement activities, and changing our basic understanding of drugs, their risks, and the marketplace itself. The most damaging of all the designer drugs are the synthetic narcotics which are hitting the streets for the first time.

Up until 1983 it was considered a regional problem—California's problem—despite deaths linked to the drugs in Oregon, Arizona, and British Columbia. Then, in late 1984, a PCP lab in Texas was seized by Drug Enforcement agents, who discovered that the lab was also manufacturing a synthetic narcotic linked to an epidemic of Parkinson's disease on the West Coast. And in 1985 Drug Enforcement agents seized two methamphetamine (speed) labs in California that possessed bootleg recipes and equipment for the manufacture of the same hazardous synthetic narcotics. These drug labs were known to be shipping their products elsewhere in the country.

Meanwhile, samples of other designer narcotics—some of them hundreds of times more potent than heroin itself—were being sold and used with cocaine. The damaging health consequences of organic drugs such as heroin and cocaine were familiar enough, but now individuals faced a new gamble. They ran the risk of smoking, injecting, or snorting a contaminated byproduct or untested derivative of a synthetic narcotic that might cause sudden death or neurological damage. Several hundred dead and the epidemic of Parkinson's disease have put law enforcement agencies, the medical profession, researchers, and, ironically, the black market itself on edge.

Until 1984, it appeared that hard-core addicts made up the majority of the dead. After the PCP and meth lab busts in 1984 and 1985, the unexpected possibility of the extremely potent and/or contaminated designer narcotics being sold as PCP, speed, and cocaine fueled a growing horror among experts privy to the information. The Centers for Disease Control (CDC) were appropriated one million dollars by Congress to continue their own investigation separate from law enforcement as the toll of death and disease continued to rise. According to an earlier 1985 CDC report:

> . . . meperidine analogs may have been mixed with other street drugs such as cocaine and phencyclidine [PCP], and users of these drugs may not have been reached by our educational efforts or may not associate the forementioned [Parkinsonian] acute or chronic symptoms with meperidine analog exposure.

By 1986, investigations of black-market synthetic narcotics were underway in Michigan, California, Delaware, Oregon, New Jersey, Texas, Louisiana, Florida, New York, and Arizona. (In 1982, the Netherlands had a similar epidemic among narcotics users exhibiting Parkinsonian symptoms.) Because of the sudden availability of the synthetics in these target areas, potential victims need to be warned and advised. But the likelihood of users paying heed to what sounds like one more "drug scare" is slim; there have been too many drug scare campaigns in the past.

The 1936 movie classic *Reefer Madness* warned users that smoking pot leads to rape, murder, and madness. A 1960s anti-LSD campaign advised all users that LSD causes birth defects. In the 1970s we were told that speed kills (challenging speedfreaks into shooting suicidal doses of methamphetamine—burning out, but certainly not dying). Ultimately, misinformation and outright lies have cost authority dearly. The price has been a loss of credibility.

With each new decade of drug propaganda, we've seen a subsequent escalation in drug use. One of the biggest mistakes in our drug abuse policy has been the failure to distinguish between hazardous and less hazardous illicit drugs. The intent here is *not* to endorse the use of less hazardous drugs but, rather, to demand honest and therefore credible drug education. Authorities on drug abuse, especially the government, tend to exaggerate the dangers of some drugs merely because they are illicit. They misclassify drugs, categorizing marijuana alongside heroin, for example. They rely on drug scare notions in the vain hope that some thirteen-year-old may believe them and decide not to experiment. But the message has been dishonest and continues to be dishonest. Kids have a keen sense for dishonesty. The authentic earns their respect. Drug education programs will be effective the day educators stick to what is known and what is unknown—the simple, undisputed *facts*. The facts are sensational enough. What the public sees, hears, and experiences will then reaffirm rather than contradict what is being taught.

That grade school and high school kids should be warned against experimenting with new drugs has never been more urgent than with the advent of these new synthetic narcotics. Let them hear not only from parents and counselors, but from the junkies, the narcs, and the emergency room doctors.

After all, it's the detectives who kick in the doors, seize the chemicals, and bust the dealers. It's the upper-income cokehead who knows what killed his friend. It's the crime lab specialist who identifies these never-seen-before drugs. It's the neurologist treating victims crippled by the products of sloppy underground chemists who can share the tragedies in vivid living detail. It's the coroner who writes up the death certificate "for unknown substance" one can chat with if still wondering just who the hell to believe.

Others "in the know"—the black-market manufacturers, chemists, and dealers—aren't quite so accessible. Some are smart entrepreneurs. Others are hack chemists getting their start cooking up sloppy batches of PCP. A rare few are brilliant research types experimenting in the black market, using drug addicts and naive consumers as their guinea pigs. To hear them talk about drugs as just another way of making money is to understand better why, for instance, purifying their product is unimportant to them as long as they have an active ingredient. Many of these amateur and professional chemists feel no responsibility for their product once it has been sold to a middleman. To hear it straight from the source is to believe it.

Whether I was in Washington talking to a Drug Enforcement Administration (DEA) official, in California talking to a convicted black-market chemist, in Chicago talking to a researcher, or sharing a cup of coffee with a suburban junkie housewife, I discovered a remarkable ignorance of and contempt for the opposite point of view. In truth, nobody believes anybody anymore, let alone listens to them.

Politicians don't listen to drug addicts.

Researchers don't listen to detectives.

Cops don't listen to users.

Users don't listen to researchers.

And, most crucial of all, no one listens to the black market.

It is a novel approach in health care drug literature to allow drug runners, dealers, and black-market chemists to speak openly about their professions and the new designer drug phenomenon. But only when you understand their motivation—the purely financial incentive and their role in the distribution network—the complete isolation from that dead addict six dealers removed or that adolescent irreparably damaged from a one-time experiment—only then will you begin to realize how much you are at risk.

Why did they talk? Some are outraged that new hotshot chemists are honing in on the territory, making millions, and killing off or crippling the clientele. They are angry because these new phantom chemists haven't "paid their dues" (serving prison time) and are "bringing the heat down on everybody else" (more law enforcement drug surveillance). An underground organization called "The Council of Cooks" to "Keep Drugs Clean" is presumably getting ready to take the matter in hand. As one drug runner told me, "We have our own way of handling business."

Between September 1985 and June 1986 I talked with researchers in Los Angeles, New York City, Chicago, New Haven, and elsewhere; I talked with coroners and toxicologists on the East and West Coasts; I interviewed convicted dealers and chemists in local, state, and federal penitentiaries; I talked with crime lab specialists in Washington, D.C., San Diego, and Sacramento.

Some of the users interviewed were celebrities who asked to remain anonymous. As one television actor told me, "It's no longer hip to toot on the set. Drugs have become deadly serious—you can lose a contract now, whereas before everyone from the director to the prop girl might be doing drugs. Everybody's still using. They're just a hell of a lot more discreet."

Drug use, as we are wearily reminded every day, has reached unprecedented levels despite more laws and more penalties. Prohibition never worked. It didn't work with alcohol from 1920 to 1933. It hasn't worked with heroin since the 1914 Harrison Narcotic Act. It's not working with pot, LSD, PCP, or Ecstasy. The demand is there and it's growing. In the last few years hundreds of unscrupulous entrepreneurs have entered the black-market synthetic drug trade. They feed on the ignorance and desperation of the user.

iv

This book is written to educate all of us about the growing availability of designer drugs and their inherent hazards: to make known the profound range of pharmacological and toxicological effects of the different drugs; to inform people so that they think twice before they snort a suspicious white powder, inject a dose of speed, or smoke a little heroin to come down off a cocaine high; and to force them, in that split-second decision, to hesitate and consider what is at stake, not because the attorney general is threatening prison terms or because the local drug counselor is challenging them, but because they know now what the chemicals are and how they react in the body. And they know the risks—death, degenerative disease, or lifetime addiction.

The doors have been thrown wide open to these new drugs. Bootleg recipes are being sold. Clandestine labs can be set up and dismantled in a few days' time. Profits are being advertised. As long as someone can make a dollar, the drugs will be sold on the street to unsuspecting consumers. For whatever reason this book is read, there will be some voice the reader will believe. But it should not be taken out of context. Not until all the experts have their say, not until the drug addict's comments are treated with the same respect as the senator's can we come to a clearer understanding of the tragedy at hand. Not until we set aside our arrogance and condescension about the opposite point of view will some of the damage being done to all of us be stopped.

With the traditional narcotics and stimulants, the effects were predictable. Now the game has become a deadly Russian roulette—it's the one shot in the arm, a few tokes off the pipe, or a half-dozen snorts—with no second chance. This book does not purport to be the final word on designer drugs. For one thing, the illicit drug trade is constantly changing. But there are sources of information and questions to be asked and demands to be made. The bottom line is this: designer drugs have become the very best reason not to do drugs.

I want to especially thank the California Narcotics Officers' Association for allowing me to attend their four-day conference and sit in on their "closed session classes." Thanks to Dean Latimer; Bob Timmons; Charles Hamm; Dr. William Langston of Santa Clara Medical Hospital; David Langness; Dr. Gary Henderson of UC Davis; Dr. Frank Sapienza of the DEA; Dr. Richard Hawks and Dr. Doris Cluett of the National Institute on Drug Abuse; Brian Leighton; Ray Wells; Jack Hamilton; Mike Murphy; Jerry Taylor; Ron Gospodarek; Dr. James Ruttenber of the Centers for Disease Control; Dr. Forrest Tennant; Dr. Darryl Inaba from the Haight-Ashbury Free Medical Clinic; Alan Clarke; Dr. Ronald Siegel; Dr. Mark Gold; Pat Gregory and Dan Largent of the DEA and State Bureau of Narcotics; UCLA for sponsoring the Designer Drug Conference; Dr. David Gorelick and all the other researchers, coroners, and crime lab specialists, the local detectives, and state and federal agents for sharing confidential information about current investigations. I would also like to thank Jeff Wack, Bonnie Hesse, Todd Smith, and Buddy Micucci for their help in preparation of this book.

Thanks to all the users who shared their experiences out of a sincere desire to help others. Special thanks to those convicted chemists and dealers who agreed to be interviewed. As one convicted chemist told me, "If my talking saves one kid's life, then it's worth it."

That is reason enough for this book.

1 Designer Opiates Arrive

As LSD and the psychedelics became the hip drugs of the 1960s, and PCP and speed the pop drugs of the 1970s, designer drugs have become the glamour drugs of the 1980s. Media coverage in virtually all of the major newspapers, in *Life, Time, Newsweek, New York, Science, U.S. News & World Report,* and the TV talk show circuit helped give the designer drug phenomenon a high profile throughout the country. The label "designer drugs," however, is both dangerous and misleading.

Essentially, designer drugs are variations of already federally controlled synthetic drugs which mimic the effects of the classical narcotics, stimulants, and hallucinogens. By slightly altering the molecular structures, black-market chemists create new, untested, legal drugs. Designer drugs also refers to "new drugs" appearing on the street such as "Crack" which are concentrated forms of already existing drugs, but are uniquely marketed for target income groups.

At the heart of one designer drug controversy is Ecstasy, fashionable as the "yuppie drug of the '80s" because of its widespread use among urban professionals and college students. Users claim it gives them confidence, happiness, verbal ease, and emotional intimacy. Its reputation in the gay community is that of a "sexy drug" replacing MDA. Psychiatrists, psychologists, and scientists were using it as a therapeutic aid for people suffering from schizophrenia, depression, and addiction.

When street abuse became widespread in 1985, John Lawn, the acting administrator of the Drug Enforcement Administration, stated: "All of the evidence DEA has received shows MDMA 'Ecstasy' abuse has become a nationwide problem and that it poses a serious health threat." At the time, preliminary studies from researchers in Chicago suggested that MDMA caused brain damage. Reports of adverse physical side effects and psychotic episodes from around the country had alarmed both the medical profession and law enforcement. In July 1985, Ecstasy became illegal and its production was forced onto the black market.

The notion of designer drugs, however, is not new to the streets. When the Feds outlawed LSD-25 in 1966, a host of designer hallucinogens and stimulants began to flourish on the black market, including MDA, MMDA, STP, and TMA. A variety of concentrated drug forms appeared, including mescaline from peyote, atropine from belladonna, red oil or hash oil from cannabis, etc. Chemical derivatives of methaqualone, PCP, and amphetamine surfaced in the 1970s. What *is* new to the streets is designer narcotics—a whole new category of drugs that mimic the classical opiates including opium, morphine, and heroin. For decades, elite crime lab specialists in Washington, D.C., speculated about when underground chemists would begin cooking up the extremely potent and potentially toxic synthetic narcotics. News came in December 1979 with the deaths of two men in Southern California.

Late 1979, two men purchased what they probably thought was heroin. One of the men was discovered comatose in a motel room. Drug paraphernalia and white powder were found near the body. The second man died in his bathroom shortly after returning home from work. Investigators could find no trace of morphine in the body fluids of either man. Not until January 1981 did the DEA special testing and research lab in Washington, D.C., identify the lethal substance as alpha-methyl fentanyl—a designer drug 200 times as potent as morphine. It was the first in a series of designer synthetic heroins that would kill hundreds of drug users. Years later it would be linked to a genius chemist operating a secret lab out of his apartment in an upper-middle-class neighborhood in West Hollywood, California.

By spring of 1980, synthetic heroin deaths began to spread from Orange County up the coast to Monterey County in California and east to Arizona.

Then, during the summer of 1982, an altogether different variety of black-market synthetic narcotic showed up on the streets: instead of killing its users, it was crippling them. In San Jose, California, forty-two-year-old George Cerrillo and his girlfriend entered Santa Clara Valley Medical Hospital suffering severe muscular rigidity and palsy. Over the fourth of July weekend, they had shared multiple doses of a powder sold to them as "new heroin." Samples of the drug were found to contain a toxic byproduct known as MPTP. Permanently crippled, both victims required medication every three hours to move, eat, or drink. The "new heroin" was intended to be a "designer" version of a synthetic narcotic known as meperidine. But the underground chemists had improperly synthesized it and created instead the highly toxic MPTP, which damages an area of the brain linked to Parkinson's disease. A lawyer-turned-chemist was known to be distributing the toxic substance from his house outside San Jose in Northern California.

At the same time, fifty miles to the south, two brothers were paralyzed after mainlining "new heroin." Within weeks, five more victims of MPTP poisoning were admitted to Santa Clara Valley Medical Hospital exhibiting symptoms of Parkinson's disease after a public television announcement was made warning users of the danger.

During the same summer of 1982, seven more overdose deaths caused by the fentanyl-series of designer heroin were reported. From the fall of 1983 to the spring of 1984, thirteen synthetic heroin overdoses were reported in the San Francisco Bay area. The killer drug was 3-methyl fentanyl, a designer heroin 3,000 times more potent than morphine and, of course, legal. It was a new "designer heroin" not seen before on the street and therefore not restricted by the federal government.

By 1984, four different designer heroins of the fentanyl series had been identified on the street, two of which were thousands of times more potent than heroin.

Urines tested from California methadone clinics suggested that more than 20% of the state's known 100,000 heroin addicts were using some form of synthetic heroin.

Between 1982 and 1985, twenty drug users were severely crippled by the toxic byproduct MPTP produced in the faulty synthesis of a synthetic narcotic derivative called MPPP. In 1985, the Centers for Disease Control identified 400 individuals who may have been exposed to the toxic MPTP, many of the victims already exhibiting symptoms of Parkinson's disease. Two deaths caused by MPTP were reported in Vancouver, British Columbia.

By spring of 1985, more than 100 deaths were linked to the fentanyl-type of designer narcotic imitating heroin on the street. The deaths had occurred in nearly every urban area of California, in addition to suburban and rural areas. Ages of the victims ranged from twenty to forty-nine years. Most were male, many were white. Unofficial reports from federal and local law enforcement agencies, researchers, and the medical community suggested that the number of deaths was grossly underestimated because of inadequate chemical analysis of body tissue and fluids. The extremely potent synthetic drugs cannot be detected with standard equipment and techniques used by coroners and toxicologists. Many of the overdoses, said the experts, go unidentified.

As a variety of designer drugs began to flourish on the black market, causing a sudden rise in overdose deaths and neurodegenerative disease, the two most obvious risks became clear. *First,* because many of the designer drugs are new drugs not tested before, their potency and selective action are unknown. *Second,* because they are produced illicitly by phantom chemists practicing no quality control, many of the substances reach the street contaminated by impurities and toxic byproducts.

The alarming increase in designer drug-related medical emergencies caught public health and law enforcement officials by surprise. Task forces at the federal and state level were formed to discuss emergency measures. Senate hearings on designer drugs fueled the growing concern. Information gathered from law enforcement, the medical community, crime labs, researchers, and abuse clinics remained widely unavailable to the general public.

By late 1985, investigations were underway in New York, New Jersey, Louisiana, Michigan, Delaware, Arizona, California, Oregon, and Texas, where synthetic narcotics suddenly appeared. Four clandestine labs making the drugs were taken down during the summer of 1985. Millions of doses were seized. However, many of the designer drugs were not yet illegal, so the chemists and the dealers could not be prosecuted.

The novel aspect of the designer drug phenomenon played up by the media was the legality of the drugs. By manipulating the molecular structures of fentanyl and meperidine, for example (controlled synthetic analgesics sold under trade names such as Sublimaze and Demerol), the designer chemist creates new drugs that mimic the effects of heroin and whose manufacture and distribution are not in violation of federal law. Publicity given designer drugs sent state and federal legislators clamoring to pass new laws making all potential analogs (derivatives) of fentanyl and meperidine illegal.

Despite the legislation, risk of prosecution for the black-market chemists and dealers remained negligible. Legislation had never deterred the amateur ghetto PCP chemists, the biker methamphetamine manufacturers, and certainly not the new breed of synthetic narcotic wizards. Publicity and prohibition did succeed in attracting more entrepreneurs to the black market. A research chemist working for Du Pont in Delaware synthesized 3-methyl fentanyl and tried selling it after reading about how much money he could make. Whereas one gram of heroin would yield approximately 200 doses, the same quantity of 3-methyl fentanyl would yield 50,000 doses.

Typically, entrepreneur chemists are attracted to the designer drug trade because it appears to be a clever, easy way to make a lot of money. The drugs can be synthesized from common industrial chemicals. There are no importation costs as with organic drugs. Some drugs are extremely potent—producing pharmacological effects identical to the classical narcotics, hallucinogens, and stimulants—and can be sold in concentrated forms that are easy to hide or disguise. The synthetic narcotics, in particular, are not detected by routine chemical analysis, making them attractive to parolees, prison populations, and a growing number of white-collar workers fearful of mandatory drug testing.

The trace amounts make it impossible to directly link a manufacturer's product to a dead user. Because the labs are virtually impossible to find without the help of informants, because the drugs are often not identified by crime labs, because the death or disease caused by the drugs may be several dealers removed from the chemists, and because of countless loophole-legalities handicapping law enforcement, the slim possibility of getting caught and serving time is a risk worth taking when balanced against the promise of big profits.

As more amateurs are lured to the black market, as PCP chemists try to synthesize the more sophisticated synthetic narcotics, as methamphetamine distributors purchase bootleg recipes for cooking up the synthetic narcotics, the potential for toxic substances reaching the streets is greatly increased. Unknown, untested hazardous chemicals are created inadvertently by faulty laboratory procedures, sloppy mistakes, and a complete disregard for quality control.

The bad batch of "new heroin" responsible for the epidemic of Parkinson's disease was the result of sloppy chemical procedure. Intending to synthesize MPPP, the chemist took shortcuts to save time. Rather than heating the product for a lengthy period of time at a low temperature, he decided to speed things up by raising the temperature. That simple but crucial mistake created the toxic by-product MPTP.

A similar mistake was made in 1976 by a twenty-three-year-old chemist who was synthesizing narcotics for his personal use. He was referred to the National Institute of Mental Health after exhibiting symptoms of Parkinson's disease. A known drug user, he had synthesized what he believed was MPPP. It was subsequently learned that he had inadvertently created MPTP through faulty chemical procedures.

Lethal mistakes can be made during the simple process of mixing the active ingredient with a common cut (diluent). Because the fentanyl derivatives are so potent, the actual dose may be as little as a microgram—less than a grain of salt. (By way of comparison, a postage stamp weighs approximately 60,000 micrograms.) Dealers along the way "step on" (dilute) the product—a technique requiring much skill and sophistication, which the street dealer doesn't have.

Illicit synthetic narcotics have spread dramatically. The drugs can be disguised to look like whatever organic heroin is currently being sold on the street, or sold as cocaine or methamphetamine to unsuspecting users. They are made to look, smell, taste, and feel like the real thing. The chances have skyrocketed for not only the addict, but the "recreational user" and that first-time experimenter— whether it's the Wall Street executive, the suburban housewife, or the junior high school student—to unknowingly sample a lethal or crippling drug.

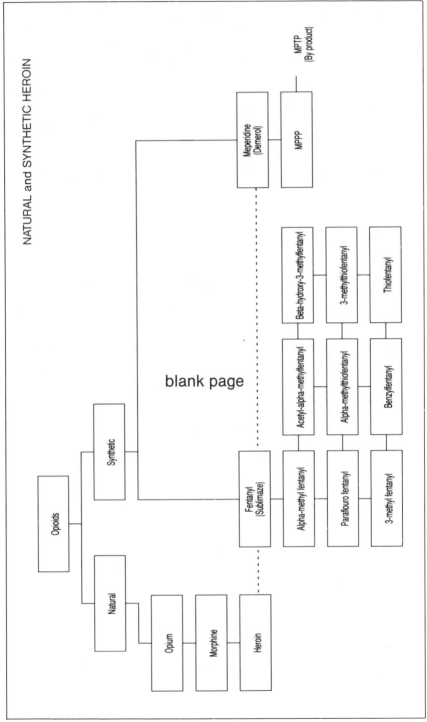

NATURAL and SYNTHETIC HEROIN

Diagram 1

2 "China White"

◆ *In early 1980, one of our recovering clients, a local jazz musician who had been in our program and was in recovery for three years and doing real well—he helped found a writers' and artists' Narcotics Anonymous program—he was doing great but he had a slip. He came into the program pinned, loaded, wanted to see me. He didn't want to detox . . . he just wanted to talk to me, and he says, "Darryl, I want to warn you—there is some China White out there—it kicks your butt! It's the best stuff out there in years." The very next week he was dead. He had died in his bathroom. Classic needle stuck in his arm . . . They couldn't find any drug in his system.*

We had clients coming in pinned to the max with this new China White . . . They gave us urines . . . no drug present . . . We sent samples to Pharm Chem, to DEA, sent them all over in 1980. They were saying these guys are getting high on milk sugar because there's no drug present. We're clinicians. We've been working with addicts twenty years. We know what it is when you're loaded. We kept pressing the issue. We sent more samples to DEA laboratories and mid-1980 the DEA lab announced that the street had created for the first time a fully synthetic [heroin] . . . for the first time in 5,000 years of opiate documented abuse in human beings.

Dr. Darryl Inaba
Designer Drug Conference, UCLA
October 1985

Counting the Dead

No one knows how many are dead from synthetic heroin. Even the experts can't agree on an estimate. It's nobody's fault, of course. Can't blame the coroners. They can't help it if their equipment doesn't test parts per billion—the trace amounts of synthetic heroin in tissue and fluid samples of overdose victims.

Can't blame the local undercover detective. His crime lab says the stuff he's seizing tests negative for all opiates and whatever the hell else he thinks it might be.

Can't blame the hypes on the street. They think they're shooting the purest Southeast Asian heroin available . . . until packs of them start dropping dead. But as one Washington official put it, "Who in Middle America really gives a damn if some San Francisco junkie dies of designer heroin instead of the real thing?"

And then the medical examiner does an autopsy on a young, upper-income, suburban, white female. Although the case exhibits classic symptoms of a narcotic overdose, the body tissue and fluids test negative for opiates. The girl's parents wait impatiently to find out what killed their daughter. A backlog of cases presses down on the medical examiner, who hasn't time to send away for more sophisticated tests. The toxicologist discovers a nonlethal trace of cocaine. Death certificate reads cocaine overdose.

Whether or not she snorted synthetic heroin thinking it was cocaine, or smoked synthetic heroin to come down off the "edge" of cocaine, or tried speedballing a synthetic heroin she thought was real "Mexican Brown" will never be known. That she died because she unknowingly smoked, snorted, or injected a homemade "designer heroin" will never be questioned. No one will discover that what killed this young woman was a designer heroin called China White—several hundred times stronger than morphine, contaminated with impurities, and disguised for sale as heroin, cocaine, or speed to its unsuspecting users.

The Public Health Service statistics will remain unchanged. The Centers for Disease Control, the National Institute on Drug Abuse, the national monitors of disease and death won't catch this one. No one will alert the local detectives. No street gossip will alarm the users. The dealers won't worry if they've "stepped on it enough." The chemist may not know the stuff is contaminated or so potent it kills instantly. He'll keep on cooking, the dealers will keep selling, and the uninitiated will keep dying.

Interview: Female. Upper income. Divorced with children. Employed. An attractive woman, despite a severe loss of weight.

Today was my day to be sick. I always plan in advance when I'm going to be sick. But I knew I had to talk to you . . . so I took just a little treat [shot heroin] this morning. [smiles] Just a little treat. When I'm sick, it's bad the first three days. After six days you think you're going to make it. After ten days the worst is over. I've been on a run maybe two months now. I don't like the people at work to know, you know. They saw me through the methadone thing—*that* I'd like to tell you about. That is the cruelest idea they ever came up with. Takes two months to get over being sick from methadone. I was violently sick two months and didn't sleep. I went back to heroin just to get clean from methadone. It's easier to get clean from heroin. They arrest you outside the clinics. It's really pathetic. Here are all these sick people. The cops know it. They're just waiting around like goddam parasites for one of the junkies to make a mistake. Believe me, it's true. I went through it all. Methadone is poison. It's ten times worse than heroin.

The first time I was turned on to heroin was through a friend. I'd known this guy for a long time. He used to come to our parties at the beach. We socialized. I never dreamed he did heroin. One night after shooting a lot of cocaine—I was very heavy into cocaine at the time—I was strung out and there was no way I was going to get any sleep and I wanted to sleep so bad. So my friend asks me if I want a snort of his stuff. I slept like a baby. That was the first time. Maybe he should have known better. [smiles]

My suppliers are friends or very good people I trust. A guy I know just bought from the alley and I told him he should have bought a couple of Snickers bars instead since all they're selling is sugar anyway. Yeah, I told him next time go eat a couple of candy bars. [laughs] Those people in the alley, they don't give a shit about the people they sell to. The people I used to buy from down in Compton were some of the most fascinating people I've ever met. I had a great deal of respect for them. They also took care of me. Where I was going was worse than Watts—very, very dangerous. I usually drove down there myself and after they got to know me, they always let me in through the gates. It is a traditional thing with them that you don't just walk in, fork over your money, and get your junk. You have to pay your respects to the family. That happened up in _____ also. There—that's the distributor, higher echelon—no gates or anything, totally respectable. We would go in and be introduced to the family members and pay our respects before conducting business. I only went along with my friend—he was buying in large quantities—I could never go there and just buy for myself. My people down in Compton were all dealer-users. The quality was a lot less down there than what the distributor was selling.

My people looked out for me. They once got very angry because another friend of mine who was also copping down there when I was there asked me to give this fellow a ride. I did and the Mexicans got very angry. They said no one was ever to get in the car with me when I was holding. They really got mad at my friend. Sometimes when I was really sick, they'd give me a balloon for free. They care about you. Once, when no one was there, I copped from one of the neighbors which otherwise is strictly forbidden. They always warned me it was a "hot" area. After I got busted, I couldn't go back there anymore. I miss them . . . Another thing about them, once they get to know you and you're a steady customer, they drop the price for you. Also, if you're sick and broke, they give it to you for free. They are good people.

The only time I remember getting anything strange was when we shot up down there and we had this incredible ringing in our ears. I mean the whole time there was this ringing. When I went back to buy again I told them not to give me anymore of that shit and they said okay. Another good sign it might be synthetic is when it burns in your arm. Just the other night at a coke party a guy told me the same thing. He was all coked up so what can you believe? You shoot up and it burns, it's sorta too late, don't you think? [smiles] Did you know there's a huge difference between the kind of people who do cocaine and those of us who do heroin? The cocaine people—the cokeheads are just a bunch of partiers. Some of them are getting bored though and starting to do heroin. The cokeheads, once they start using, they'll buy any shit off the street!

Not too long ago, a dealer sold me some stuff and told me not to cook it. I always cook my Persian with a little lemon and always cook my Mexican. I don't like it when they tell you not to cook it. I don't trust it. A friend of mine died not long ago. He bought some bad stuff. I don't know who he bought it from. Somebody must have been with him. You need an introduction before you can just go buy from somebody.

I asked my doctor the other day if he could check me for AIDS. I told him I was in a high-risk group. He asked what difference would it make. I said that I want to know if I'm going to die in five years because I want to have a lot of fun before I go. He didn't think I should know and I don't.

One of the problems with shooting up with men—I've observed this on several occasions—they have this thing, it's sort of a macho thing. They like to watch you get things ready. They watch me cook it up and fill the syringes and then when everything's ready, they always have to be the first to shoot. And they almost always make me wait while they go into the bathroom and comb their hair or whatever the hell. But I've learned my lesson. I just sit and wait very patiently and I never say a word. I know the game they're playing. Another thing, I am a very neat, clean person. I like to have my own [syringe]. I put my name on my needle and label theirs with their name. But it never fails, after we first shoot up, they always reach over and take mine! I think to myself, Jesus Christ, can't ya read? This one's mine. This one has your name on it. They're all alike.

I sometimes get sick from cotton fever. That's when you save your cottons for when you run out and then use what's left in them. You get bad chills and fever. I think it's because one of the tiny cotton strands goes into your veins. When my people heard that I was saving my cottons, they thought that was really pathetic and gave me a free balloon.

A friend of mine, he's gay, got a new boyfriend who's an alcoholic. He can really pick 'em! I don't drink, period. I am also a vegetarian.

Malibu, California
September 1985

Gathering the Evidence

Three days after Christmas 1979, two men in their thirties mainline synthetic heroin. Both arrive dead at Anaheim Memorial Hospital in Southern California. The first man is discovered comatose in a motel room and ticketed DOA at the hospital. The second man returns home from work and promptly dies in his bathroom. Needle, syringe, and a white powder resembling heroin are found near the bodies. Both drug samples contain lactose—a milk sugar used to dilute heroin. Both are packaged in balloons, the way heroin is sold on the West Coast. To the utter bewilderment of investigators, chemical analyses of blood and tissue samples of the victims test negative for all narcotics and other drugs of abuse.

Within twelve months, a dozen similar cases are reported in California and Arizona that exhibit the classical symptoms of narcotic overdose, including pulmonary edema and evidence of sudden death. No drug can be detected in the corpses or in residue from samples confiscated at the site. A suspected link in several of the deaths is that the drug used has been called "China White"—a term previously used only for pure Southeast Asian heroin. A number of informants, however, insist that the drug being sold to users is "synthetic heroin."

Here's the twist. Word gets out in the media that this new synthetic heroin "China White" is killing addicts. Hypes watch the news. People stop buying China White. Meanwhile, a few dealers really are selling China White—the really pure Southeast Asian heroin. Now they can't *give* it away. So what do they do? The poor slobs dye it brown and sell it for less money as "Mexican Brown"! From what I gathered, a couple of DEA agents up in Northern California got the bright idea to call this synthetic heroin "China White." All they accomplished was mass confusion.

Crime lab specialist
Los Angeles Sheriff's Department
September 1985

By late 1980, the DEA's Special Testing and Research Laboratory in McClean, Virginia, had samples of the suspicious white powder to analyze. The largest sample the researchers had to work with was 200 milligrams, from which they extracted approximately one milligram of active ingredient—barely visible to the naked eye. They examined it with a nuclear magnetic resonance spectrometer, which locates the positions of atoms in a molecule. It took three months of research to positively identify the substance as an analog (derivative) of fentanyl known as alpha-methyl fentanyl.

In addition to China White's appearance on the West Coast, the DEA identified powder samples of alpha-methyl fentanyl taken from a clandestine lab in New Jersey in May 1981.

I can tell you one curious bit of information . . . Way back in 1979—I got the exact date in my records—I keep a book of inquiries that agents make of me when they call and ask me questions about clandestine labs . . . an agent called back around October 10, or thereabouts . . . and gave me a list of chemicals and the name of an individual and said, "What can you make from this stuff?" And I said, "Well, gee, I don't know." I thought about that for a long time. And for months I didn't know what could be made from it . . .

What happened next . . . we got a case of the first fentanyl analog we'd ever seen: alpha-methyl fentanyl out of Borrego Springs [first death] and that took three months to identify . . . We had it done at Special Testing . . . Well, it turns out that to make that you can use at least some of the chemicals that were on that list that was given earlier. Until that identification, those were two separate instances. The only thing that tied them together was that I realized, hey, this one chemical could be useful in making this other thing—this alpha-methyl fentanyl. Furthermore, on that original list in 1979, he wanted a lot of nitric acid and I never did figure out exactly what he wanted that for . . . We knew where he wanted to purchase these chemicals . . . They were cooperating with us, retailers and wholesalers both . . . we got an invoice from the chemical company . . . that's how we *knew* the list of chemicals.

Well, when we went into his place [six years later] we found a lot of records, invoices, and things like that. And I found *that* invoice. With *that* date on it! I said there was a lot of nitric acid on that original order and I didn't know what that was used for . . . When we got this lab, I figured it out! It was many steps removed from the actual fentanyl analog and was used early on to make a key part of the intermediate used in the final product . . . It took six years for that to come clear to me and what I'm getting at . . . I do believe, he is the person who is responsible . . . that he is the guy that started the whole thing.

DEA chemist
West Coast
January 1986

Between 1979 and 1981, twenty deaths were directly linked to alpha-methyl fentanyl after a series of elaborate "catchnets" and sophisticated tests. Dozens, perhaps hundreds, of other deaths slipped past the experts.

Approximately 200 times stronger than morphine, alpha-methyl fentanyl was the first of ten fentanyl "designer heroins" to appear on the black market. The DEA placed it into Schedule I of the CSA (Controlled Substances Act) effective September 22, 1981. Until a drug is classified as a controlled substance by the federal or state government, it remains legal both to make and to use.

At one of the funerals for the hypes that overdosed [in 1984], one of the dealers attended. A friend of the hype who died, an addict himself, accosted the dealer at the funeral and accused him of selling bad shit. The dealer said it was great stuff and gave the hype a free sample. They found him dead in his car.

DEA agent
Northern California
October 1985

Alpha-methyl fentanyl is a simple derivative of fentanyl. Fentanyl itself is a synthetic narcotic used in more than 70% of all surgeries in the United States. Its chemical structure is different from heroin and morphine, but it possesses identical pharmacological and toxicological effects. Almost any alteration of the fentanyl molecule will yield a potent narcotic.

Fentanyl was first introduced in 1968 as an intravenous analgesic-anesthetic (painkiller) under the trade name Sublimaze. It is approximately 100 times more potent than morphine, has a rapid onset of two to three minutes and a short duration of action of thirty to sixty minutes. By rearranging, adding, or snipping off groups of atoms from the fentanyl molecule, the underground chemist created a new legal drug that mimicked heroin's euphoric rush and could forestall withdrawal sickness. The new "designer heroins," however, were untested and contaminated. Each new derivative to appear on the streets differed in potency, euphoric effects, toxicity, and length of action. The effect on the human body was anyone's guess. The unsuspecting buyers were the first test guinea pigs.

We had maybe 15 cases we suspected were fentanyl-related overdoses that we sent to UC Davis for the more sophisticated chemical analysis using GC-Mass Spec. We had every reason to believe they were fentanyl-related because they involved known heroin addicts, the typical paraphernalia . . . We were amazed to find all tests negative for narcotics. We were even more amazed when [Dr. Gary] Henderson came up empty as well. It's a good possibility this may have been an altogether new analog so potent—in nanogram quantity [billionths of a gram], it escaped all detection . . . Then again, there are any number of adulterants or contaminants that could be lethal, and we simply haven't the time to test for them all . . . If there's adequate evidence but not complete, it's better to establish what seems obvious . . . We do quantitative analysis but we don't need a lethal dose in the body fluids to confirm overdose . . . In some cases we'll find alcohol along with narcotics. More often we find cocaine. Any number of combinations can give you the characteristic massive pulmonary edema . . . We've had so many screen negative for the fentanyl we had no choice but to write them off as unknown substance.

Toxicologist
San Francisco
September 1985

After the first deaths were reported in 1979, eight more were confirmed in 1980 and 1981 as synthetic heroin traveled in California from Orange County and San Diego County up the coast to Monterey County then across to Arizona. Seven more deaths were reported in 1982. Eleven deaths tested positive in 1983 as the designer heroins shot north to Santa Clara, Sacramento, and the San

Francisco Bay area. In 1984, forty-nine deaths were linked to fentanyl derivatives, two of them in Oregon. Nine of those deaths occurred within days of one another in August, all in the San Francisco Bay area.

When police found Anthony Gilbert Flores behind a Menlo Park hamburger joint just before midnight June 30, rigor mortis had already set in. The 36-year-old self-employed carpenter was still standing beside the open driver's door of his Chevy truck, leaning over the seat. The needle was still in his arm. Instead of heroin, police suspect, Flores got fentanyl, a powerful synthetic narcotic up to 7,000 times as potent as an equal weight of morphine.

San Francisco Examiner
August 29, 1984

Between the fall of 1983 and spring of 1984, 3-methyl fentanyl appeared on the streets. It is approximately 3,000 times stronger than morphine, 1,000 times stronger than heroin. It was blamed for more than a dozen overdose deaths in the San Francisco Bay area. As mentioned before, the active dose is a microgram—a postage stamp weighs approximately 60,000 micrograms. It was scheduled under the Controlled Substances Act by the DEA effective April 25, 1985. Recipes for the drug were discovered in a fentanyl lab seized in June 1985, in West Hollywood, California. A second chemist in Delaware was arrested in December 1985, trying to sell a large quantity of 3-methyl fentanyl.

A hundred more deaths were estimated for 1986 as the designer heroins made their appearance in New York, New Jersey, Florida, Michigan, Delaware, Oregon, and Arizona, with large seizures made in Louisiana and California. Law enforcement learned of one shipment to London in 1985.

You hand out pamphlets on the dangers of synthetic heroin to the hypes in Palmer Park, and I guarantee they'll turn around and use it for toilet paper when they take a shit in the bushes.

Lieutenant
Los Angeles Sheriff's Department
September 1985

Dr. Gary Henderson, professor of pharmacology at the University of California at Davis, has been researching the fentanyls, tracking the deaths, and testing for fentanyl in body tissue and fluids of suspected overdose deaths sent to him from across the country. He has compiled a variety of statistics and hypotheses, including the following: The fentanyl series of designer heroins have killed in suburban areas, semirural areas, and nearly every urban area of California; ages of the victims range from twenty to forty-nine years; the majority are male and white. Dr. Henderson has said that the overdose deaths reflect only a small fraction of those who are using the drug.

The old-time hypes use only their own syringes. They buy from the same dealer with a couple of back-ups if he goes dry. They test their stuff in small quantities. They do not buy anything that looks suspicious. They won't be the ones dying from the synthetics. It's the new users. The young punk kids.

Narcotics detective
San Francisco Police Department
October 1985

Fentanyl killed my friend. He was using for eleven years. Successful businessman. His habit cost him $2,000 a week. He had gone to see a new supplier. Just that one time, he just couldn't wait. He died instantly. It had to be synthetic. He had incredible tolerance.

Cocaine dealer
West Coast
September 1985

Studies conducted at methadone clinics in Northern California show that 10% of the clients tested had used fentanyl derivatives either knowingly or unknowingly. A clinic for heroin addicts in Marin County, north of San Francisco, revealed that 65% of its clients were using fentanyl.

The victims are not coming out of hard-core urban addict populations but are the "chippers," the "recreational users," the novices. A new class of upscale junkies—those "social users" who imagine themselves different from addicts because they don't shoot up—appear to be most at risk, smoking and snorting heroin in combination with cocaine, a variety of other drugs, and alcohol.

Everybody and I mean everybody in the punk rock scene is doing heroin. What happens is—you get these kids coming in from Fullerton or what-the-f— suburb and they want to be with what's happening. They got their punk haircuts—their mohawks or what-the-f—, and they don't fit in with the rest of the kids back where they came from. They see people look like them in Hollywood and cuz Hollywood's "where it's happening" and everything and these people are shooting heroin, well, hey, they're cool, they're with what's happening in Hollywood. They look like them and they do what they do. They go back home and they say, "Hey man, I'm with it, you assholes don't know what's happening." What's happening is shooting heroin.

Drummer
Punk rock band
January 1986

By November [1985], [Boy] George had graduated from cocaine to heroin, which he was using on a fairly regular basis. On one occasion, he acquired some "really synthetic smack," according to Jane, and became violently ill. For several days he was so sick he couldn't leave his bed. Once he recovered, though, he started smoking and snorting the drug. He apparently never used a needle. "He's never injected, ever," said Fat Tony. "When someone thinks of a junkie, they always think straight away of a syringe. That's got nothing to do with it. Snort it, burn it, whatever, it's all the same thing. I don't think he understood whatsoever how heavy a sort of a hold it would get on him. At that point he thought he could stop it at any time."

Michael Goldberg
Rolling Stone
August 28, 1986

After the flurry of overdose deaths in Northern California, Dr. Darryl Inaba described the victims as white, upper middle class, educated— and dumb about drugs.

We are on to a dealer—major dealer in town working out of a nightclub dance place selling cocaine cut with heroin. Lot of upper-income kids in their twenties. The girls are the worst. Our informant tells us they keep coming back for more because it's the best coke in town. They don't even know they're junkies.

Narcotics detective
Hollywood, California
January 1986

What's on the Street

When supplies are low on the street, the synthetics make their entrance. Availability, price, and needing a fix—there's your scenario . . . For every bust on imported heroin, it's one step easier to sell the synthetics.

Cocaine dealer
West Coast
January 1986

Street names for fentanyl derivatives that have been sold to unsuspecting users include "China White," "synthetic heroin," "fentanyl," "Mexican Brown," and "Persian White."

When we questioned one of the dealers, he told us most of the buyers were lied to. They were told it was real heroin when they asked if it was fentanyl, synthetic, or China White. He told us a lot of addicts were asking too.

Federal agent
Northern California
January 1986

Physical Properties, Adulterants, Packaging

The fentanyls have been sold in powder form. Pure white is sold as Persian White. Light tan is sold as China White or as synthetic heroin and fentanyl. Light brown is sold as Mexican Brown—the brown color acquired by carmelizing the lactose or using a dye.

In [Derrick's] place [fentanyl lab] we found some dyes—brown dyes and we could conjecture why he had them there. I know why. I think he was going to mix it with this stuff [confiscated fentanyl derivatives] and try and make it look like Brown Mexican heroin.

DEA chemist
San Diego, California
January 1986

Textures of the fentanyl derivatives vary from finely powdered to coarse and cake-like, depending on the cut. The fentanyls have been diluted with large amounts of lactose or sucrose (powdered sugar) or mannitol (mild baby laxative). They have been mixed with heroin to augment poor quality. They have been mixed and used with cocaine. They have been adulterated with quinine (disguises the taste), and diphenhydramine (an antihistamine).* Since the active ingredient is exceptionally small, less than 1%, it is unrecognizable by color, odor, or taste. Some samples have a medicinal or chemical odor.

We arrested this dealer and he's got two kinds of fentanyl mixed together with a dash of heroin for good measure. Now what the hell's he thinking about? Both the analogs were still legal. If he's prosecuted, it'll only be for

Narcotics detective
Southern California
October 1985

---

*The toxic actions of morphine-like narcotics involve the release of histamine into the circulation which in turn causes nausea and vomiting. Fentanyl does not trigger release of histamine. Dealers adulterating the fentanyls with diphenhydramine increase the risk of excess sedation.

We estimate, in our program, the designer opiates comprise
about 10% of our patient population [use] and that may be a
very conservative estimate because what we're finding out in
1985 is that the designer heroins, the new synthetic heroins, are
being used to augment low quality heroin. When you die, they
don't find the synthetic—they find the other.

Dr. Darryl Inaba
Designer Drug Conference, UCLA
October 1985

Synthetic heroin is very much available on the streets. It is in
high demand because it is more potent. The user is looking for
a better rush. I know the dangers but the street users don't.
We have no educational pamphlets to warn them of the
hazards.

Recovering addict/drug counselor
Sherman Oaks, California
September 1985

Some addicts have been advised that the best way to test suspicious
samples is to check for water solubility, since fentanyl compounds
are water soluble and will dissolve without heating. However, to test
for water solubility is impossible because street samples are 99.9%
diluent. The active ingredient is measured in micrograms and is
unidentifiable. A single dose of 3-methyl fentanyl, for example,
contains five to ten micrograms, or one-quarter to one-half of a
grain of salt.

I don't know if the people . . . got the material in premea-
sured dosages or not because I never got it that way. When I
got it, it was like a big bag—ten pounds all cut. Let's say it
was a tenth of a percent of the active drug ingredient . . . All
the rest is lactose and maybe some other junk . . . But that
doesn't mean you can't say a person's still got an overdose
because, while the percentage may have been right, who's
going to sit there and monitor how much this guy shovels in
his spoon when he cooks up? If he shovels too much in there,
I don't care if it's a tenth of a percent or not, it's still going to
kill him . . . In other words, you could take a teaspoon full of

a tenth of a percent or you can take a grain of salt of a pure thing and the little grain might kill you and the teaspoon might not because it was cut so much.

> DEA chemist
> San Diego, California
> January 1986

Synthetic heroin? Never heard of it. I wait 'til somebody else at the party shoots up. If he's okay, then I do mine.

> Punk rocker
> Hollywood, California
> December 1985

Packaging includes balloons, plastic bags, and foil packets—typical of the West Coast heroin market. Synthetic heroin was only recently seen on the East Coast sold in glassine envelopes with an identifying trademark.

We got one dealer selling a kit with ten balloons of synthetic heroin and a bindle of cocaine for an antidote! That way they just die wired to the gills!

> DEA chemist
> Northern California
> October 1985

Black-Market Chemists

There are three types of clandestine chemists. First are the amateurs, who pick up their expertise watching others cook. They usually start out synthesizing PCP because it's easy, then pick up new techniques and bootleg recipes from the street and in the prison system.

The second type are the pros, chemists employed in the public and private sectors who enter the black market because they can't earn enough money legitimately to satisfy themselves. They are most often college educated with a fund of laboratory experience and access to research material.

The third type are the wizards—the designers of new drugs—who may or may not have any formal training. The following profiles of chemists linked to the manufacture of designer heroin have been gleaned from news sources and investigating detectives and agents from the East and West Coasts. For purposes of discussion, the "Whiz Kid" is the wizard, the "Goof-Up" is the amateur, and the "Altar Boy" is the pro.

The Whiz Kid

> ". . . world-class . . . a mysterious genius."
>
> *Dallas Morning News*
> May 1985
>
> ". . . mastermind."
>
> *New York Times*
> March 1985

Derrick. Born 7-7-43; white; two years' college chemistry, independent study at UCLA; prior arrest record for manufacturing and distributing PCP and other controlled substances. Derrick was arrested April 13, 1986, by DEA agents and West Hollywood Sheriff's Department detectives at his apartment in West Hollywood while operating a clandestine laboratory suspected of manufacturing fentanyl derivatives (synthetic heroin).

He does extensive research in the scientific literature. He works very hard. He took an end molecule and built it up himself doing various reactions. Imagine an orange-flavored chocolate cake with vanilla frosting. Say you have eggs and a dab of lemon for starters. Now come up with every step in the process and all the ingredients to make that exact cake. That's sort of what he did. He is an excellent organic chemist, but he's no good in quality control. We were finding a soupy mixture of impurities in his products. He always made the same sloppy mistakes. We could recognize his work from the telltale impurities. We could usually tell if it was his or not . . . I'm sure he's gotten a lot of ego gratification knowing he's stayed one step ahead of us all this time. He's what I'd call the

research type. Not your typical PCP street chemist. He's one
of a kind. A very rare individual.

Dr. Frank Sapienza
DEA chemist
Washington, D.C.
November 1985

Derrick was indicted April 14, 1986. He was accused of manufacturing sixty pounds of synthetic heroin since 1983 and faces twenty-
six charges including conspiracy and attempt to defraud the FDA,
failing to register a drug with a federal agency, and distributing a
drug without a label or a list of ingredients.

He's a timid little hippie. He served eighteen months of a two-
or three-year sentence at Soledad for selling an uncontrolled
substance as a controlled substance. He sold alpha-methyl
fentanyl to an undercover L.A. County deputy sheriff and said
it was heroin. *That* convicted him. "Sales in lieu of." At
Soledad he met two inmates that later worked as dealers for
him in the Fresno and San Jose area. He never sold directly to
them. He only sold to one main distributor, a Mr. Q—. Mr.
Q— sold to the two dealers and then they had their own street
dealers. At one point we were following Mr. Q— on Hwy. 99
thirty-five miles south of Fresno. He had $90,000 in cash in the
trunk of his car and a loaded .44 revolver . . . In [Derrick's]
lab we found formulas for 3-methyl fentanyl. We don't know
if he gave the formulas to anybody. In one transaction, he sold
eight pounds of synthetic heroin to Mr. Q—. According to one
of [Derrick's] dealers, the product was usually stepped on four
or five times before it reached the street and if it wasn't
stepped on at least three times, you could guarantee an
overdose. He told us there was a meeting in December 1984 or
January 1985 between Mr. Q— and the two top dealers to
discuss the overdose deaths. He said they never contacted
[Derrick]. Mr. Q— denies meeting with the dealers but he's
just trying to cover his own little ass. They met to discuss a
change in potency and how in hell they could control it.

Federal narcotics agent
Northern California
December 1985

Derrick had formerly been arrested in July of 1985, after DEA agents seized several pounds of synthetic heroin valued at approximately $3 million. He was released because the drugs were not illegal at the time.

When we raided his apartment [April 1986], his lab was set up and cooking. The whole place stunk like chemicals. He was at the sink dumping chemicals down the drain. We unscrewed the sink traps and confiscated the chemicals! He was very low-key. Didn't want to talk. I started feeling woozy and I asked him, "Am I gonna die breathing this shit?" He says, "I'm sitting here, aren't I?" After we confiscated the unknowns and a bunch of amphetamines, codeine and a PCP analog called PCE, I said, "[Derrick], we're sending you back home." He said, "Where's that?" I said, "T.I.—Terminal Island." He shook his head and said, "The food's no good there anymore. Not since Reagan's cutbacks."

He had five different bank accounts. The first one had over $300,000. We had to hand everything over to the Feds before I could check the others. He's sort of a wimpy little guy, fashions himself quite the ladies' man. He had girlie magazines all over the place.

Narcotics detective
Hollywood, California
February 1986

Derrick was asked about the deaths linked to synthetic heroin. He maintained that the doses were kept uniform, and described an elaborate chemical procedure. When asked if a user could tell the difference between synthetic and real heroin, he replied, "No." When asked what advice he might give users, he said with a smile:

"Just say no."

The Goof-Up

Wait until all these amateurs fooling around with PCP and methamphetamine try their luck with the fentanyls. Then you'll start seeing fireworks.

Clandestine lab agent
Northern California
October 1985

Harold. Late forties; black; Ph.D.; educated Southern California; prior arrest record for manufacturing PCP. Harold was arrested July 1985 at a house in North Hollywood while operating a clandestine lab believed to be synthesizing fentanyl derivatives. Desmethylfentanyl was confiscated (thought to be intermediate stage of 3-methyl fentanyl). Desmethylfentanyl was not illegal at the time of Harold's arrest, and he was released from custody.

Although Harold is college-educated, he is more representative of the amateur PCP and speed chemists who make the transition into the more sophisticated synthetic narcotic chemistry via bootleg recipes.

[Harold] may have a Ph.D. but I wouldn't call him too bright. We walk into the place and it's not even ventilated! The whole lab was set up and he's sitting there crying like a baby, drinking beer and playing cards. This is the same guy who blew himself out of a cabin and once out of a boat while cooking PCP.

DEA clandestine lab head
Southern California
September 1985

All I know is if we'd raided the guy when he was end-stage and opened the place up, set up fans and blown the stuff out the windows, we'd have wiped out a neighborhood.

DEA chemist
Northern California
October 1985

[Harold] was leagues behind [Derrick] in sophistication. He declined to talk to us . . . He was sick too. He'd been breathing that methylacrylate. The paramedics checked him out pretty thoroughly. Showered him off on the street there with water . . . I don't know if he was seriously sick or just wanted to complain that he was sick. He didn't want to talk . . . His lab was set up and operating and it was a piece of junk too in the sense that it wasn't carefully controlled and he had run a reaction in the bathtub! He had chemicals all over the place—in the air, on the carpet—what a mess.

DEA chemist
Southern California
January 1986

The lab was heavily armed—sawed-off shotguns . . .

Clandestine lab agent
Los Angeles
September 1985

[Harold] is the perfect example of a PCP man making the move into synthetic narcotics. He's got to worry more about blowing himself up or just killing himself breathing in the drugs than he has to worry about the law. He got burned at the last lab he blew up, which I was told was a fentanyl lab.

Clandestine lab agent
Los Angeles
September 1985

The Altar Boy

Howie. Early thirties; white; Ph.D., University of Wisconsin; research chemist for E. I. Dupont de Nemours & Co., Wilmington, Delaware. He was arrested in December 1985 and charged with carrying out a drug-trafficking scheme through confidential post office boxes, classified ads, maps, buried drugs, and money.

Howie is not your typical clandestine chemist. As a legitimate research chemist he may be leagues ahead of underground chemists in knowledge and experience, but also incredibly naive about the black market, its distribution system, and the contacts needed to put himself in business.

According to an affidavit filed in U.S. District Court in Wilmington, Howie allegedly sent an anonymous letter to a co-worker at Dupont offering $10,000 if the co-worker could line up a dealer to pay $900,000 in gold in exchange for extremely potent, legal designer drugs—synthetic heroin. In letters held as court documents, Howie is alleged to have talked about future drug deals for which he could prepare new, unregulated, and completely legal designer drugs just by altering the structures. "The only problem is that we have no way of knowing how potent they are until somebody uses them. I can keep an unlimited supply of the fentanyls available, despite the slow, lengthy preparation . . . These dealings are going to make us very rich."

He said he first got the idea after reading an article in *Chemical Engineering News.* He had underlined direct quotes from DEA authorities stating that the designer drugs were simple to make, had a huge return on the investment, and were extremely potent. From the time he first got the idea, it took him two months working with Dupont chemicals during regular work hours to synthesize 3-methyl fentanyl. Knowing nothing about street trade, he advertised in the interoffice mail hoping to find a distributor or dealer. He had an altar boy background. December 16th, the DEA busted his lab at Dupont and confiscated [approximately] three ounces of 3-methyl fentanyl. He guaranteed buyers he could make any uncontrolled analog they wanted. He probably will serve the maximum sentence—15 years.

DEA agent
Delaware
January 1986

The co-worker alerted Dupont security, who turned it over to the DEA. An elaborate scheme involving maps and buried ammunition boxes and classified ads in the *Wilmington News Journal* ensued. Before picking up a $260,000 installment on the drug deal, Howie provided one ounce of 3-methyl fentanyl in a buried ammunition box with instructions that each ounce of the drug should be cut with 3,000 pounds of lactose. One ounce of 3-methyl fentanyl cut for the street is estimated to equal 62 pounds of pure heroin worth $28 million on the street.

There are a lot of chemists working in the marketplace earning
$20,000, $30,000, maybe even $40,000 a year. The idea of
making half a million bucks for a couple months work starts
looking better and better the more they read about it in the
newspapers. They'd be smart to just keep quiet about all the
money can be made—the people doing all the advertising.

Convicted chemist
State penitentiary
West Coast
September 1985

I don't think you're going to give somebody an idea like that
[synthesizing heroin] who wouldn't have gotten the idea some
other way anyway. Besides, everybody knows there's a lot of
money in drugs.

DEA chemist
Southern California
January 1986

Effects on Users

The fentanyls, like the opiates, primarily act on the central nervous
system and the gastrointestinal tract. They produce analgesia—relief
from pain. They produce euphoria and drowsiness. They also
produce varying degrees of respiratory depression, constipation, and
muscle rigidity.

My hypes are telling me they don't like it. Slams 'em down so
they can't do anything. Normally, they fix, maybe watch
football on TV. But this new synthetic puts them out. What
the hell fun is that? Right now in the industrial areas and the
ghetto you can't *give* that shit away. Why the hell do you think
they're browning it up to look like Mexican?

Narcotics detective
Southern California
December 1985

The most common route of administration is intravenous injection. Smoking and snorting the fentanyls was presumably growing in popularity as word traveled of their high lipid solubility, making them smooth and easy to snort.

Controlled studies have shown that addicts perceive fentanyl subjectively as having heroin-like effects. In California we have found many individuals enrolling in methadone treatment programs who have only fentanyl in their urine upon admission, yet are convinced they use only very high-grade heroin. Therefore, when pharmacologically equivalent doses are used, most users probably cannot tell the difference between heroin and the fentanyls.

Dr. Gary Henderson
Senate Hearings
July 1985

The rush or euphoria experienced after injection, inhalation, or snorting is dependent on dose and route of administration. The effects tend to be more intense. Some addicts complained of an intense rush and an overwhelming, short-acting high that "they might just as well have slept through" and was "over and done with before you could blink." One addict complained of a burning sensation in his arm upon injection—a symptom associated with Demerol-type derivatives known to be contaminated.

Addiction liability is extremely high, since the fentanyls produce both tolerance and physiological dependence following repeated use.

The plasma life of the different fentanyl derivatives is unknown. Plasma life is the approximate length of time the drug saturates the receptor sites in the brain. (See Narcotics and the Brain, below). At the end of the plasma life, the addict must "fix" or begin withdrawal symptoms. The plasma life of heroin is four to six hours. When using the shorter-acting fentanyls, an addict may have to fix more often to forestall withdrawal.

Anyone that's been through the heroin game pretty much knows you only get high for the first six days [months?] . . . and that's the only high you get. After that, you're paying dearly to just stay well. You never get high again . . . Now I never been through the heroin thing, but I did it all. I did the brown, I did the white, I did the synthetic—the fentanyl— which is ungodly strong. There was this tiny cocaine spoon no bigger round than this [1/2 inch] . . . and to be just barely showing at the top. I just did one side and could barely keep myself awake. That's how strong it is. I snorted it. Did heroin in combination with cocaine a couple times but I'd never allow myself to do just straight heroin. Cuz I know it's supposed to be *real good* . So I wouldn't allow myself to have that pleasure in case it did try to get its hook in me. No chance.

Convicted manufacturer, dealer
State penitentiary
January 1986

The most acute toxic effect of the fentanyls is respiratory depression. Degree and duration of respiratory depression for the different fentanyl derivatives on the street is unknown. Following 200 micrograms of fentanyl given intravenously, maximum depression occurs within five to ten minutes and normal respiration returns within fifteen to thirty minutes.

At Paula Hawkin's hearings [Senate subcommittee hearings on designer drugs, spring 1985] two hypes were asked by the Senator if they were not truly scared by all they had just heard and seen. The one fellow said it was good to know all of this but, in fact, when they see an ambulance going for an OD, they follow it to find out where the OD was getting his stuff because it was probably really hot stuff. He said the experienced junkie can handle it, it's the novices who die.

Dr. Frank Sapienza
DEA chemist
Washington, D.C.
November 1985

Depression of respiration is caused by direct actions of narcotics on brain stem centers, which sense carbon dioxide levels in the blood. The lack of oxygen that follows severe respiratory depression may lead to a drop in blood pressure. Blood pressure may eventually become so low that cardiovascular collapse occurs and death results.

> Heroin addicts [are] always looking forward to their next fix and always having a lot of fun. Methadone people take their fix once a day and then got nothing to do the rest of the day. The heroin guy has his blood levels going up and down at a regular rate and it's all quite exciting, going from semi-withdrawal to instant ecstasy and a nod, into normality, and into semi-withdrawal—sniffles, cramps, goosebumps, getting anxious, and bang, back to instant ecstasy. It's a lot of fun. Methadone is boring. [With heroin] you're masturbating your whole endocrine system.
>
> Former speedfreak
> New York City
> November 1985

Fentanyl produces a decrease in heart rate of up to 25%, with a parallel drop in blood pressure of up to 20%. The effects of the black-market fentanyl derivatives on heart rate and blood pressure are unknown. That the derivatives are more potent than fentanyl itself suggests more intense effects on the cardiovascular system.

Why Are Users Dying?

The exact cause of death in fentanyl-related "overdoses" is debatable. Many experts believe it is the potency of the drug. Three indicators that potency may be the culprit are:

1) the physical symptoms of the deaths, most especially the massive pulmonary edema and the sudden manner in which the user dies (the needle still found in place);

2) the fact that several times deaths occurred in groups in the same areas at the same time, indicating that users—both addicts who can tolerate extremely high doses as well as novices—have taken the same batch of designer narcotic; and

3) the size or quantity of dose. Since doses are in microgram amounts, it is easy for an extra grain or two to triple potency.

You would have to do an outstanding job of mixing. In the
lump of powder, a tenth of a percent is fentanyl and the other
99.9% is something else, probably lactose . . . even if you did
a good job mixing, the stuff still might settle because they
might have different densities or other different physical char-
acteristics . . . That is a very difficult job to get something
adequately mixed and then even more difficult to make sure it
stays that way.

DEA chemist
Southern California
January 1986

Whether or not massive pulmonary edema and suddenness of
death are symptomatic of overdose has been controversial for years.
Some researchers suggest that the cutting agent used to dilute the
active ingredient may be the cause of death.

If there's strychnine or quinine . . . used as a cutting agent
and we aren't informed of this, we aren't going to run tests for
it. There isn't the time.

Toxicologist
Northern California
November 1985

In 1966, at a meeting of the Society for the Study of Addiction in
London, Dr. Milton Helpern, former chief medical examiner for
New York City, was asked the cause of massive pulmonary edema:

To my knowledge it is not known why the pulmonary edema
develops in these cases . . . This reaction sometimes occurs
with the intravenous injections of mixtures, which, as far as is
known, do not contain any heroin, but possibly some other
substance. The reaction does not appear to be specific. It does
not seem to be peculiar to one substance, but is most
commonly seen with mixtures in which heroin is the smallest
component.

In a paper published on September 15, 1966, in the *New York State Journal of Medicine,* Dr. Helpern suggested that death may result from sensitivity to the material used as a diluent to the heroin:

> Unexpected acute deaths may occur in some addicts who inject themselves with heroin mixtures even though others who take the same usual . . . dose from the same sample at the same time may suffer no dangerous effect. In some fatal acute cases, the rapidity and type of reaction do not suggest overdose alone but rather an overwhelming shock-like process due to sensitivity to the injected material. The toxicologic examination of the tissues in such fatalities where the reaction was so rapid that the syringe and needle were still in the vein of the victim when the body was found, demonstrated only the presence of alkaloid, not overdosage.

Dr. Helpern stated that some of the mixtures killing users "do not contain any heroin" and in some cases "only the presence of alkaloid," and that "the syringe and needle were still in the vein." Although at the time Dr. Helpern was trying to make a case for overdose caused by alkaloids or cutting agents, the evidence suggests an even more astounding possibility: that a designer heroin may have been on the streets as early as the 1960s but was never detected.

Contaminants of the synthetic heroin may also be killing users. The active ingredient may be diluted properly but, because it was not purified in the clandestine lab, carries dozens of other byproducts that individually or in combination could kill the user. These byproducts and contaminants are often new to the scientific literature.

> There are things in some of those mixtures that we will never know the identity of . . . I'll never know, that's for sure, and I've worked on them [confiscated fentanyl derivatives] for three or four months. There's a lot of information we're lacking. Two key areas. One is that not very much research has been done on the physiological response of the pure drugs themselves. Two, no research has been done on any of the byproducts . . . A third point is that no research has been done on the synergistic effects of two of these things in combination. One of the samples [seized June 1985]—you couldn't count the

number of different components! But I did count fourteen
primary components. One major product. Thirteen other
things that weren't intended to be there. No research has been
done on the other thirteen in terms of what they'll do to the
body . . . or what would happen if you had all these things in
combination—I mean, who would *do* that?!

DEA chemist
San Diego, California
January 1986

Another consideration as to why the designer heroins are killing
their users is the synergistic effect of multiple drug use. How deadly
can a combination of synthetic heroin and cocaine be? A study of
cocaine deaths in major cities of the United States indicates that one-
quarter of those deaths showed evidence of heroin. If so many users
are dying from the combination of heroin and cocaine, one can only
conclude that the risk runs even higher when designer heroin is
substituted (whether knowingly or not).

The following, then, are all possibilities as to why users are dying:

—the potency, which is often several hundred times stronger
than heroin;

—the high percentage of quinine, diphenhydramine, and other
street adulterants used to cut the microgram doses of
fentanyl derivatives;

—the untested byproducts and contaminants created by sloppy
black-market chemistry; and

—the synergistic effects of cocaine, alcohol, and other drugs.

Narcotics and the Brain

Numbers of overdose deaths? A hype is a hype is a hype. He's
gonna shoot up anything he can get his hands on. Tell him
you'll sell him something that will give a good rush, the boy
will jump on it. When's the last time you saw a sick hype with
the shakes and snot all over his face? They get desperate

enough, on their knees, they'll shoot speed if you give it to them. No little info on the hazards of designer drugs is gonna interest a hype. Not when the boy's sick.

Narcotics detective
Hollywood, California
October 1985

In 1973, specific receptors for opiates in the brain were discovered. The natural opiates produced by the body were themselves discovered in 1975. They were called endorphins, a class of neurotransmitters. In general, the endorphins are the body's natural way of dealing with stress. Norepinephrine is another natural neurotransmitter, and it reacts to painful, panic- or anxiety-provoking stimuli. In the October 1985 issue of *Equinox,* David Kline, in his report entitled "The Anatomy of Addiction," presents one theory describing what might be happening in the brain:

> When someone uses heroin, the brain is swamped with artificial endorphins. The user experiences euphoria, a physical soothing that masquerades as a superior sense of well-being, and a stoicism toward the gloomier side of life. In the presence of all that heroin, the body's self-regulating endorphin system believes itself redundant and shuts down. If the heroin is abruptly stopped, the firing rate of norepinephrine increases because there are no natural endorphins to inhibit it. The result is the symptoms . . . in detoxifying addicts.

Those symptoms include runny nose, tearing, sneezing, irritability, insomnia, loss of appetite, abdominal cramps, pains in the bones and muscles of the back, excessive sweating, nausea, tremor, increased heart rate and blood pressure, and diarrhea, all leading to weight loss and dehydration.

Dr. Roy Wise and Michael Bozarth of Montreal's Concordia University Center for Studies in Behavioral Neurobiology have done studies involving another neurotransmitter called dopamine, which, like endorphins, is responsible for what people experience as euphoria and pleasure (and has been implicated as a player in narcotic withdrawal and cocaine psychosis). Those studies indicate that both heroin and cocaine activate the same reward systems in the brain. Cocaine prolongs dopamine action by blocking its reabsorption, and heroin causes dopamine to be released initially. (See diagram 2 on page 65.)

With depletion or dysfunction of the body's natural supply of endorphins and dopamine, an individual's ability to deal with everyday stress is dramatically impaired as is his natural reinforcement system that allows him to experience pleasure. The body has its own way of telling itself when it has done something good. Thus we feel pleasure after waking from a good night's sleep, eating a hearty meal, or comforting a child. After chronic use of an artificial "reward" like heroin or cocaine, the body's natural reinforcement system partially shuts down, causing everyday pleasures to be devoid of joy. Life can become unbearably gloomy without an artificial replacement for the diminished action of endorphins and dopamine.

There is no effective cure for opiate addiction. Furthermore, growing evidence suggests that irreparable damage can be done to the brain's receptors from a single injection of either too much or too potent a designer heroin (including all of the fentanyl derivatives). The damage occurs from the devastating bombardment of receptors by neurotransmitters.

Short-term solutions are available. Some experimental nondrug therapies for treating withdrawal have shown positive results. Meanwhile, the value of such organizations as Narcotics Anonymous cannot be underestimated.

The Law

In late 1985, the U.S. Senate voted to ban "designer drugs." The legislation, sponsored by Senators Strom Thurmond, (R.—SC) and Lawton Chiles (D.—FL), was approved by a voice vote without debate and sent to the House. Part of that legislation reads as follows:

> Any person who knowingly or intentionally manufactures with intent to distribute, possesses with intent to distribute, or distributes a controlled substance analog for human consumption shall be fined not more than $250,000, or imprisoned not more than fifteen years, or both. Any person who knowingly or intentionally possesses a controlled substance analog all or part of which substance is intended for human consumption shall be fined not more than $25,000, or imprisoned not more than one year, or both.

First time I did China White I thought it was cocaine. I
snorted it, got the sweats, and vomited. Did it again later on.
Then I went to prison. Long story. In prison you take
anything you can get. I did some stuff I *know* was bad.

White female, mid-twenties
Los Angeles
December 1985

In California, State Assemblyman William Filante introduced
Assembly Bill 2401 in January 1985, which controls all analogs of
the parent drug fentanyl. It was signed into law by the governor on
September 27, 1985. As of January 1986, no black-market manufacturer, chemist, dealer, or distributor of the fentanyl series of synthetic
narcotics had been convicted of trafficking illicit synthetic heroin.

Law enforcement efforts against designer drugs have been
limited. According to DEA, only four clandestine designer
drug laboratories have been immobilized in this country, one
in October 1984 in Brownsville, Texas; one in April 1985 in
San Diego; and two in June 1985 in North and West Hollywood, California. The designer drug phenomenon could revo-
lutionize the way drugs are used and sold in this country.
Designer drugs are manufactured in clandestine laboratories by
phantom chemists. The cost of manufacturing designer drugs
is only a fraction of the cost of smuggling heroin or cocaine
into this country, and the profits to be realized are much
greater. Consequently, the potential exists for organized crime,
which controls the heroin and cocaine markets, to enter into
the designer drugs area, in both the production and distribution ends.

Senator Lawton Chiles
Senate Subcommittee Hearings
on Designer Drugs
July 18, 1985

The Big People [organized crime]—hell, they're like corporations, I mean the big f—ing people who'd make the decision,
"Okay, do we go into these analogs [derivatives] or do we stick
with trusty old Smack?" Somebody who'd make a decision
like that would do it methodically. They are very conservative.

Because they got this problem: if they *do* start going into
analogs, if the analogs are so easy to make, then by god, they
are going to have all their little fly-by-night people to worry
about. How do you fit that into this network they got now,
incredibly unwieldy and complicated? Taking the poppies in
Afghanistan and getting them out through f—ing Calcutta and
getting the morphine base to Europe, cooking it up into heroin
in Europe. Moving it here through god knows how many
channels . . . There are millions of people going to be put out
of work. Lot of relations back there in la Campagna gonna be
put out of work if this shit does take over the market . . .
Believe me, the country is full of chemists. The country is full
of people who know a little bit about chemistry. Just enough
about chemistry to possibly make this shit if they could get
their hands on the glassware and stuff and if you have a lot of
people asking for it.

We've got the best Smack [here] in New York City . . . don't
get any variations. Everything's very dependable. Mob has its
hand on everybody has anything to do with heroin here. There
aren't any pirate independents trying to muscle in. When that
happens here, they get killed.

Dean Latimer
New York City
November 1985

I've stayed away from fentanyl for two reasons. In 1974, a
friend of mine, a fellow chemist, had synthesized an extremely
potent fentanyl analog. It was a couple thousand times more
potent than heroin. He was blotting one and two microgram
doses. His best friend overdosed on it. My friend was so
shaken, he quit the business. Just up and quit and left for
Europe. I never heard from him again. I was there at the time.
It was very depressing. Second reason is simple: too much
work. The handful of chemists out there synthesizing fentanyl
analogs are usually research nuts. The bottom line is money,
of course. They all do it for the money.

Convicted PCP chemist
California state penitentiary
September 1985

The Designer Heroins

The designer heroins listed below have been seized and identified by law enforcement. One seizure from a clandestine lab in 1985 contained substantial quantities of six of these derivatives. Two other seizures in California and Louisiana also contained substantial quantities of four of these derivatives.

Alpha-methyl fentanyl

First illicit fentanyl derivative to appear on the streets. Sold as China White or synthetic heroin. Approximately 200 times more potent than morphine. Shorter-acting than heroin. Associated with twenty narcotic overdose deaths during 1980-1982. DEA placed it into Schedule I of the CSA effective September 22, 1981.

Paraflouro fentanyl

Appeared about the time alpha-methyl fentanyl was placed on the restricted list. Potent narcotic equivalent to heroin. Little is known about the compound. Not seen before in the scientific literature. Disappeared quickly from the streets. Classified as a Schedule I drug.

3-methyl fentanyl

Between the fall of 1983 and spring of 1984, this derivative appeared on the streets. It has been associated with over a dozen overdose deaths in the San Francisco Bay area. It is approximately 3,000 times stronger than morphine in the body. Presumed to have the same duration as heroin. The active dose is a microgram. It was scheduled by the DEA effective April 25, 1985.

Acetyl-alpha-methyl fentanyl

Approximately ten times more potent than morphine in rats. First identified in August 1983 in Modesto, California. Thirteen other samples identified in 1984 and 1985.

Alpha-methylthiofentanyl

Over four kilograms seized at a clandestine lab in California. Samples found since 1984 in both California and Louisiana—most recently in June 1985. It is estimated to have a longer duration of action than fentanyl and is between 450 and 600 times more potent than morphine.

Benzylfentanyl

Identified in more than twenty-five drug evidence submissions from the San Diego area between January 1982 and June 1985. At least twenty-four fentanyl-related overdose deaths reported in the same area during same period. It is an intermediate in the synthesis of fentanyl and is, itself, an active morphine substance with an analgesic potency about one-tenth that of morphine administered to rats.

Beta-hydroxy-3-methylfentanyl

Analgesic potency in rats estimated to be about 300 times and possibly 1,500 times that of morphine. Four different evidence submissions identified in California in 1985. Over four kilograms confiscated at clandestine lab in Los Angeles in 1985.

3-methylthiofentanyl

Estimated potency is 1,000 times stronger than morphine administered to rats. Confiscations made in California and Louisiana in 1985.

Thiofentanyl

Four drug evidence submissions in 1985. Approximately five kilograms of material—two of the samples seized at clandestine lab. Approximately 175 times more potent than morphine.

3 "Crack"

◆ *The attraction of the freebase high is the initial rush, which subsequent tokes rarely recapture. This hardly keeps anyone from trying, and with the comedown in such strong contrast to the rush, an attempt is usually made to maintain the short-lived high by consuming repeated doses of increasing amounts. This often results in binges lasting from several hours to several days. It is very common among freebase users to attempt to balance the extreme high with some type of depressant. Once relaxed, it is even easier to consume freebase in mass quantities.*

David Lee
Cocaine Handbook:
An Essential Reference

Coke Dealers Compete

Cocaine has glutted the black market. Despite the Reagan administration's five-year crusade spending unprecedented sums of money, using the most sophisticated technology, stepping up manpower, and permitting the use of Navy and Coast Guard ships, Black Hawk Army helicoptors, and the Air Force in its war against cocaine, the drug has never been more plentiful, cheaper, purer, or more widely used.

Law enforcement isn't what's worrying black-market dealers. The competition is. Cocaine entrepreneurs have resorted to new marketing techniques and packaging in order to stay competitive in the industry—an industry to rival *Fortune 500* companies as annual sales of cocaine reach $60 to $70 billion.

And, like other industries, the black-market trade in cocaine is not immune to supply problems. As the glut of crude oil sent oil prices plummeting, so has a soaring supply of cocaine drastically reduced prices on the street. The cost of a kilogram of cocaine (2.2 pounds) has been driven down from $50,000 wholesale to $32,000 and dropping.

Tough competition has inspired suppliers and dealers to market their product in much the same way as legitimate businesses—through product improvement and more attractive packaging. Cocaine is being "redesigned" to sell to a more demanding, ever-changing marketplace.

Enter "Crack" — the cheapest, most potent, most addictive form of cocaine to hit the streets. The dealers have shrewdly figured out that they can sell more product and attract more buyers if they freebase the diluted street cocaine they are selling. Ten dollars of snort cocaine for a lousy couple of snorts cannot compare to ten dollars of freebase worth three incredibly potent "tokes" from a cocaine pipe giving what one Crack user described as "a jarring, shocklike, agony of bliss."

Although Crack is often no purer than the street cocaine from which it is processed and contains nearly the same percentage of adulterants and impurities, it feels purer because smoking the concentrated alkaloid gives a more immediate, intensified rush. This happens because the smoke is absorbed into the bloodstream through the lung tissue—the most direct route to the brain. The profound rush is instantly experienced and quickly disappears. Snort cocaine, in contrast, is absorbed much more slowly through the mucous membranes in the nose, circulates to the brain several minutes later, and gives a less effective high which lasts twenty minutes or more.

Crack has been "designed" for the consumers who are willing to try prefreebased cocaine but unwilling to freebase it themselves because they either don't know how or are frightened by the prospect.

It has been designed for users who have built up a tolerance to regular snort cocaine and want something stronger without having to inject it (because of widespread fear of AIDS).

It has been designed for the pseudo-connoisseurs who imagine they are buying the purest product (although most cuts — with the exception of sugars — can be easily freebased through with the cocaine).

It has been designed for the consumer with $5 to $15 of disposable income—millions of experimental and occasional users who have not had, until now, the opportunity to become compulsive users because they either couldn't afford to, were afraid of the law, or had no access to freebased cocaine.

Most crucial of all, Crack has been designed for the user who is unaware of its devastating effects. The one thing dealers like best about their new, improved product is its extraordinarily addictive power. In dollars and cents that means repeat business. The customers are hooked until their money runs out. The market push has been directed at the young and the ignorant.

By May 1986, the "CBS Evening News with Dan Rather" reported that Crack had become a national problem. The 800-Cocaine Hotline reported 600 Crack-related phone calls per day. By June 1986, *Time* magazine had the National Cocaine Hotline estimating that one million Americans in twenty-five states had tried Crack! Crack had become the "Pied Piper of American Youth," according to one House Representative as testimony about Crack was heard before panels in both the House and the Senate. Crack, in a matter of months, had earned rank as a national security issue. Whether or not the exponential estimates of Crack users could be backed with corroborating evidence—emergency room reports, law enforcement arrests, users checking into health care facilities for treatment—was irrelevant as the country devoured news of Crack-smoking dens, instant addiction, dead sport heroes, and teenage Crack-whores. The dealers couldn't have bought themselves livelier publicity.

As one catchy advertising campaign asked: "Who could ask for anything more?" Crrrrrrack.

> **Interview:** Thirty-one-year-old white male. Electrician and part-time musician. Unmarried. Extremely agitated throughout interview.

> I'm not a druggie and I'm not all strung-out. I am a very creative individual and consider myself a real health nut. I have a lot of sinus problems and every time I used to sniff cocaine I'd start sneezing like you wouldn't believe. Imagine someone taking a ten-inch feather and putting it up your nose and twisting it around up in your sinuses—that's why I moved to freebase. I'm sort of a purist anyway and that pharmaceutical cool smoke was so clean and pure and never gave me aftereffects. I've been doing it for a

year and a half. I was first introduced to freebase two years ago by a good friend from Ohio. He showed me how to cook it with baking soda, though I'm a natural in the chem lab anyway. When he arrived, he just went down to the local head shop and bought everything we needed—all the glassware and tiny wire mesh and everything . . .

I almost always buy a half-gram [of street cocaine] at a time, base it myself with baking soda and distilled water, and then—and I'm the only one I know who can do this—make a quarter-gram last two hours. I'm a real connoisseur—I take little hits off the pipe and then get busy with whatever I'm doing all night long, like working on electrical projects. I get a lot of freelance work at night fixing anything electrical. I like to smoke a little all night long while I'm working. Just little tokes. Not like these other people who suck in a huge amount and then it's all gone. I know all about the dopamine depletion and I think, wow, they must really be f—ing themselves up.

I always use certain weights and measures—I'm very exacting when I base my coke because I keep a running percentage on exactly how much cut I'm getting in my stuff [confuses salt loss with street cuts that base through]. I always cook in a test tube. I buy only the best cocaine hydrochloride—usually 80% purity. The quality sometimes varies—I know how much it's cut but it isn't something you complain to the dealer about. I sometimes report to other buyers the percentage of cut. Sometimes I'll buy maybe four grams and cut it some more myself and sell it and then I figure fifty to a hundred bucks profit and a half gram maybe for me. Though lately I've noticed on reflection that I'm smoking up more than just the profits.

I know all about the compulsion and that's why I only do maybe a half gram every two weeks or so . . . But it's also why I'm quitting. I don't like the compulsion thing. When you see you have only a few tokes left on the pipe, it's incredibly depressing because you really want to keep going. When you're smoking—I don't use water with my waterpipe because I think it sucks up some of the residue—there's condensation on the glass and in that film is some of your base. So when I get near the end, I really turn up the blue flame and burn that residue which is good for a few more smokes—we call it hitting the resins.

But so the main reason I'm quitting—I quit three weeks ago and have only done it once since then—is because of this compulsion thing, the money and my lungs—I've got this steady ache I think I can clear up if I quit now. I know it's the basing because I don't smoke. I don't want to see a doctor because I really don't want to see what my lungs look like. I see the deposits on the glassware.

I was keeping tally the last few months. In February to maybe, um, well a month or so ago, I noticed on my blackboard I'd spent $485 [averaging a half gram every few days]. I call it melting the ice. Watching all that money go. I told my dealer, "Hey you guys, let me know if you see me around here too much . . ."

One thing I noticed was that when I planned projects—like I always say, "Ok, I'm going to buy a half-gram and do it tonight while I learn the lyrics to that song or play my guitar." But I usually never stop with the pipe and then pretty soon it's 4:30 A.M. and I'm laying there shaking wide awake wondering about getting to work at 8 A.M.

I smoke pot maybe twice a day and do acid when I can get it. I've done a lot of acid. Like I said, I'm a creative person and I'm into different realms of abstraction.

I've got a terrific analogy for what freebasing is really like. Imagine you are on an island and offshore about a dozen yards is this orange-pink haze that is glowing and extremely enticing. So you walk out into that cold, dark water and you swim a ways to get near that glow and you're out on the edge of it and it feels so good and so warm, but it moves away a little. So you swim out into deeper water and this time you get even closer to the center and it is so incredibly seductive. But now it's moving a little faster out into the ocean and you swim harder trying to keep up and you're getting farther and farther away from shore. That's how with the first few tokes you feel pretty good and then with a deep toke you are near the center and it's so exhilarating but you come down and keep wanting more. Pretty soon you are way the hell out in the cold black ocean and you're faced with keeping up swimming harder toward that warm, wonderful, glowing haze just out of reach or turning back and swimming miles back to shore in that dark, cold water.

San Fernando Valley, California
May 1986

Coca Leaf vs Freebased Cocaine (Crack)

As early as 1965, it was discovered that freebase cocaine is much easier to smoke than cocaine HC (hydrochloride) because it is more volatile and decomposes less when heated. Freebase is precipitated from a water solution of cocaine HC by adding an alkaline substance such as baking soda or ammonium hydroxide. It can then be either filtered out or dissolved in ether which is removed through evaporation. The base is then most commonly smoked in a glass water pipe layered with fine mesh steel screens that trap the drug as it melts.

The coca leaf itself, from which the freebase alkaloid originates, has been used by South American Indians as a stimulant to ease physical labor at high altitudes. Its purpose and utility for the Indians are in striking contrast to the highly concentrated freebased cocaine smoked in our society purely for pleasure and usually at the exclusion of all other activities.

"I went once and stayed four days," said a 17-year-old from Queens who, together with two friends, brought $200 to a Manhattan base house and smoked it in less than an hour. To get more Crack, she said, she had sex with the operators of the base house and other customers. In those four days, she slept little, ate nothing, and occasionally took short walks outside. "When you run out, that is just what you do," she said. "With me, I didn't care because it is just about getting high."

New York Times
May 18, 1986

When you're basing, everyone is in this zombie stupor watching and waiting for the pipe in total silence. Maybe somebody might mumble something but eyes are on whoever is controlling the dope—how much cocaine he's going to share with the rest of them. It is the most anti-social drug I know.

Businessman
Former freebaser/dealer
California
July 1986

The eastern sloping valleys of the Andes mountains have been the main source of erythroxylum coca leaf cultivation. The highlands of Bolivia and Peru have been the center for coca chewing since the time of the Inca Empire.

The Indians consume coca leaf by chewing its leaves with less than a pinch of the lime found in plant ashes or calcinated seashells. The leaves are chewed until softened so that stalks and strings can be removed. Lime assists in the release of the alkaloid. The amount used is critical to taste and the amount of alkaloid released. Emphasis is on the sweet, aromatic flavor of the leaves, which are sucked, not chewed, once a proper mixture with the lime and proper moistening is achieved.

In contrast, freebased cocaine is the extraction of the coca alkaloid cocaine taken to an extreme. It can be done by either of two processes:

1) Cocaine hydrochloride is the salt form of pure cocaine and is soluble in water. "Freebase" is the alkaline form of cocaine. When an alkali like ammonium hydroxide is added to a water solution of cocaine hydrochloride, the cocaine (base) is freed from the HCl molecule. Using a solvent like petroleum ether, the cocaine base may then be separated from the water by filtration or extraction. This is extremely dangerous because of the highly volatile chemicals.

2) Dealers and distributors of Crack practice a second, less dangerous process. The cocaine hydrochloride is dissolved in water. Sodium bicarbonate is added to make the solution alkaline. The mixture is then heated until all the water has evaporated. The waxy base that remains contains the added alkali and, in the case of street cocaine, a nearly equal percentage of the original adulterants and cuts used to dilute the cocaine hydrochloride. Thousands of synthetic and naturally occurring drugs used to cut the cocaine hydrochloride convert to freebase and are "based through" along with the cocaine itself.

Whereas the coca leaf wad is sucked in the mouth for approximately forty-five minutes—the time it takes to walk two kilometers uphill with a pack, which is referred to in Peru as the cocada (a standard unit of time and distance measure)—freebased cocaine is smoked and bypasses the blood-brain barrier, giving the user a euphoric "rush" within seconds and lasting approximately five minutes. This exhilarating high is then followed by an agonizing comedown haunting the user into compulsive consumption.

> The very first time I did freebase, it literally brought me to my knees. The first rush is absolutely the best bodily feeling you can get on earth. It is heavenly. But it's just that one time. I spent three months basing—always doing more and more trying to get that same first rush again . . . I quit after basing one weekend from 10 A.M. Saturday until 1 P.M. the next day non-stop. It hit me all of the sudden what a scumbag I'd become. I was taking ten milligrams of Valium to come down. Sleeping all day and basing all night. It's the same feeling you get buying on credit. You experience this reward without deserving it. I had no control in my life and business. I *was* a scumbag.
>
> Businessman
> Former freebaser/dealer
> California
> July 1986

> Here's where the merchandizing of cocaine comes in . . . If you're going to take snort coke and try to sell it in increments of $15, you would have such a little teeny-tiny bit of it—less than one line of it—nobody would pay $15 for less than one line . . . You'd be able to snort it once, maybe get two snorts, and that would be your whole $15 gone. But freebase—you get these little teeny-tiny chunks and they're really potent. Every time you smoke it, you only get one inhalation, but by god, it is a *rush*. Instant rush! It's worth fifteen bucks to get three instant freebase hits rather than a couple of relatively gentle snorts.
>
> Dean Latimer
> New York City
> November 1985

The coca leaf's primary use by South American Indians today is as a stimulant that eases labor and as a folk medicine.

Coca appears to maintain the teeth and gums in a good state of health; it keeps teeth white. The leaf is rich in vitamins, particularly thiamine, riboflavin, and C. An average daily dose of coca leaves (two ounces) supplies an Indian of the High Sierra with much of his daily vitamin requirement. Coca appears to have a beneficial influence on respiration, and is said to effect rapid cures of altitude sickness. It also rids the blood of toxic metabolites, especially uric acid. Indians say that regular use of coca promotes longevity as well. According to Indian tradition, coca was a gift from heaven to better the lives of people on earth.

Andrew Weil
"The Green and the White"
The Coca Leaf and Cocaine Papers

In dramatic contrast is freebased cocaine, which is used purely as a pleasure drug to the exclusion of all other pleasures, including food, sleep, sex, family, and friends.

Have you ever been in a room full of basers? It's awful. Like you're not there. It's only them and it. *It* is all that matters to them. I'm what they call a social baser. I take my two [hits] then pay for everyone to have their share. I go over by myself and enjoy it in a corner . . . Left my wife because she was basing all the time. Got so where we couldn't come home unless she had enough to last her. Then [she would be] going out all night looking for it. She based her own [street cocaine]. She did it every way, but decided baking soda was the best . . . She came [to my workplace] and made a terrible scene the other night and started with the alligator tears demanding money. Hadn't seen her in over two months . . . She's a prostitute now.

Gourmet chef
Los Angeles
June 1986

One big difference between sniffing and smoking is that you'll sniff with friends or maybe your girlfriend. But freebasing you save for when you're alone. I never wanted to share it. Not even with a girlfriend. It makes you very greedy and selfish and pointed inward.

Electrician, musician
San Fernando Valley, California
May 1986

I inhaled it, and when I blew it out I got that ringing in my ears—wiinnnnngggg, real high . . . I call it getting a ringer . . . It's like enjoying an all-league climax . . . All I wanted to do was freebase . . . I had a habit that was costing me $1,500 to $1,800 a month . . . I had to see the jailhouse door slammed shut . . . I had to see my family shy away from me, the wife I doubt I could live without grow disgusted, the mother and father I love and respect grow ashamed. I had to see players I considered close friends go through the same deterioration . . . their talent blowing away.

Don Reese
NFL defensive lineman
Sports Illustrated
June 1982

Whereas coca leaf chewing has religious, medical, social, and cultural significance with no recorded adverse physical effects when taken in the customary fashion, smoking freebased cocaine is an illicit activity that destroys lung tissue, causes severe damage to brain neurotransmission and brain receptors (see Effects on Users, below), and stimulates an unquenchable addiction.

What's on the Street

Street names include "Crack," "Supercoke," "Freebase," "Rock," "Roxanne," "Baseball," "Gravel," and "Base."

Physical Properties, Packaging

A light brown or beige pellet or small rock sold in clear plastic vials or the regular amber glass coke vials.

"I've seen it as white as piano-key ivory."

Former speedfreak
New York City
July 1986

Approximately 300-500 milligrams per vial (unless you buy more rocks). Two or three inhalations per rock when smoked. Average $10 to $15 per rock per vial.

Business cards "Crack It Up" and "Buy One, Get One Free" handed out by the more enterprising dealers.

I don't know what the hell they're talking about all this news stuff about the big bucks these dealers are making. They say they're making double and triple the money. No way. Take a half gram of cut street coke say for fifty bucks. Okay, I base that down to maybe six little rocks. I sell each of those rocks for maybe ten bucks each cuz that's what they say they're selling it for on the East Coast. That's a ten-dollar profit for all the hassle. Big deal. It sure as hell isn't double your money. What a bunch of hype.

Drummer in rock band
Hollywood, California
May 1986

Adulterants

Mannitol (mild baby laxative)

Lactose, sucrose, dextrose, etc. (sugars)

Caffeine

Amphetamine, methamphetamine (speed)

Inositol (B vitamin)

Quinine (causes ringing in the ears, headache, nausea)

Lidocaine, procaine, tetracaine, etc. (synthetic local anesthetics)

Ephedrine

Phenylpropanolamine

All the local dealers learn how easy it is to do and since coke is
so cheap it becomes economically irresistible to sell it this way.
What they'll do is take the regular snort cocaine that they get
all cut, usually cut down to 20% or 30% . . . with lidocaine or
any of the 'caines . . . and base it using baking soda—it's real
simple, safe, ya don't blow up. You base the 'caine right
through with the cocaine . . . it's only 40% cocaine but it's
freebase. Now everybody *thinks* cocaine freebase is pure.
That's not true. If you use this baking soda, you get *cut coke*
. . . It's economical since it's cut that deeply to sell it real
cheap . . . That brings cocaine into the reach of school kids,
not to mention housewives, busdrivers, everybody who never
used to do cocaine except for real special occasions now can go
get a little bit of cocaine in that freebase. Instead of ten or
fifteen bucks on the Lottery every week, they put that ten or
fifteen bucks to cocaine.

Dean Latimer
New York City
November 1985

I figured maybe some cuts based through because I noticed on
my wire mesh [in the pipe] there's a black tarry build-up and
it's probably dextrose or some other cut that's turning to
carbon. I'm always having to change the wire mesh layers.

Electrician, musician
San Fernando Valley, California
May 1986

Who Is Using Crack?

By January 1986, Crack had been reported in California, New
York, Iowa, Maryland, Michigan, Florida, Alabama, and Washington state. By June the media claimed it was all over the country. It
was said to be most popular throughout inner-city ghettos, replacing
snort cocaine as the drug of choice among young blacks, Hispanics,
and street-level white coke junkies.

Rumors of its rapid spread into middle- and upper-income suburbs
remain unconfirmed because few statistics are forthcoming from
national health care centers and law enforcement agencies. The
sudden notoriety of Crack illustrates a peculiar phenomenon involv-

ing illicit drugs and the media. When a previously little-known drug, however dangerous, attracts media attention, it is given widespread publicity. The public becomes curious, wants to know more, and people experiment. A demand is created and supplies increase.

Dr. [Arnold] Washton first heard about Crack early this year from two 17-year-old patients at Stony Lodge, the suburban psychiatric hospital. Both reported that they had snorted cocaine for a while, but did not become compulsive until they tried Crack—doubling, tripling and quadrupling their use, missing school, stealing from their parents and lying to their friends. These were kids from from upper-middle class families in Scarsdale and Mamaroneck. Kids with no history of addiction or psychiatric illness. They were in the top half of their class, college bound and they were addicted almost instantaneously. They were rendered completely dysfunctional by Crack in a two- or three-month period.

New York Times
November 29, 1985

Yeah, I been startin' to see the cars with the outta state plates comin' into the neighborhood . . . the white kids are startin' to get hip to Crack. Pretty soon they be as f—ed up as the kids down here. Cause that's who Crack's f—in' up the worst is the teenagers, both guys and girls.

User
High Times
November 1985

The average age of callers reporting use of Crack to the Cocaine Hotline is seventeen years. Of a random sample of 200 callers, 28% claim to have been rapidly addicted to Crack. Of these, one half were under the age of 25. Adolescents who fall into the experimental group of users and are not considered high risk for compulsive use are said to be trying Crack once or twice and finding it irresistible.

You might think you're cool and can handle anything without gettin' f—ed up . . . But don't even try Crack *one time*. That's some negative shit.

User
High Times
November 1985

Law enforcement and health care officials worry about the young naive users who think they can try Crack just once for kicks if the opportunity arises. They remember the cavalier attitude from the 1970s responsible for widespread abuse of cocaine despite publicity concerning its addictive and damaging properties. That attitude prevails today with more new users trying cocaine than ever before.

We have a strange waiting room at the Haight-Ashbury—lots of colorful people: men dressed up as women, punk rockers—the spikes coming out of their heads, bald heads with swastikas and spiders tattooed on them, but the strangest creature in that waiting room in the past few years has been Grandma and Grandpa—well dressed and well kept—they're coming in because somebody turned them on to cocaine . . . it's permeated every level of our society, no matter how you want to measure it.

Dr. Darryl Inaba
Designer Drug Conference, UCLA
October 1985

Crack Factories

Crack is processed and packaged on the East Coast in what have come to be called "Crack factories." The street cocaine powder, already adulterated and heavily diluted, is freebased into tiny pellets using baking soda, then packaged—one to three pellets per miniature plastic vial.

It pays as a distributor to freebase it, because it makes you sell your brand quicker than the next guy.

User
High Times
November 1985

"Rock cocaine" is the West Coast version of Crack and has been doing a brisk business for the last five years. The clever merchandising of East Coast Crack hasn't yet caught on as West Coast users pay more money for larger chunks of the freebased coke weighing a quarter-gram and up. A June 1986 *Time* magazine article reported that 55% of recent cocaine arrests in New York City were Crack-related and two-thirds of 2,500 coke arrests in Los Angeles in 1986 involved Rock cocaine.

> A lot of people was afraid to base because of what happened to Pryor and to other guys in the neighborhood . . . Plus it was like some people didn't really know how to do the process and didn't want to waste no coke to find out. So like the dealers came up with a way to process the coke for basing before they sold it. That way they could get a lot more people strung out behind basing because that's where the major money is.
>
> User
> *High Times*
> November 1985

"Basehouses" and "Crackhouses" have been compared to heroin shooting galleries. Apartments, hotel rooms, and abandoned buildings have been sights for freebase binges. By May 1986, a new upscale-type Crackhouse began to appear on the East Coast (Los Angeles has had a variety of Rock houses for years): reinforced steel doors, full-time armed security guards, sales of Crack through drawers in a reinforced wall, and quiet music and folding chairs for the users.

> After about 1:00 or 2:00 A.M. when everything else closes, everybody goes down to this so-called art gallery downtown [Los Angeles]. There's a back room where you can smoke base and they provide the pipes. Lot of people just snort out front. I went there thinking to make a few extra bucks. I told this really cute girl I had a lot of coke if she knew anybody wanted some. So she brought over one guy and I took his money and said I'd be right back and if he didn't trust me I was gonna leave my girl with him—I'd just met the chick! So I went to the back, bought some coke—not the base, and sold it to the guy for some free snoots.
>
> Drummer in rock band
> Hollywood, California
> May 1986

Effects on Users

The attraction of Crack is the initial euphoric rush. The smoke is drawn into the mouth and absorbed into the bloodstream through the lung tissue. This is the most direct route to the brain and the most effective means of absorption. The effects are instantly and overwhelmingly felt but are experienced for a short period of time. The initial "kick" is felt within ten seconds and the high rarely lasts beyond ten minutes. It is followed by a devastating comedown, an acute depression that causes the user to crave another hit. The positive/negative reinforcement is as pronounced in individuals with nonaddictive histories and personalities as with individuals having a propensity toward chemical dependence.

I haven't done freebase in months. I now get more charged up after working all day and doing a fine piece of work. It charges me up as much as coke did. Or a great dinner. My wife and I have become gourmet cooks. We water-ski and it's just plain fun and healthy. There are a million things to do that are healthy and fun. Working in the garden—*staying busy* . . . the people we know still doing coke have empty lives, they're trying to fill a void. They are just plain unhappy people and they become more and more unhappy because they're spending all their money and dreading having to face the morning . . . they get high to give themselves the illusion that their lives are exciting and they are successful, beautiful people . . . But, Jesus, you know, I try not to ever think about freebasing, you never forget that wonderful feeling. Just thinking about it, I start sweating, my heart beats faster. The sound of the torch will set me off! I totally agree you're a hell of a lot better off not knowing what you're missing.

Commercial illustrator
West Coast
July 1986

Snorting or smoking cocaine can kill in different ways. Cocaine overstimulates the cerebral nervous system, which causes convulsions that lead to respiratory collapse. Cocaine increases blood pressure which—depending on the physical condition and ability to handle stress of the user—can result in a stroke. Cocaine causes heart attacks by constricting coronary arteries that supply oxygen to the heart.

Freebase binges are likely to bring on respiratory failure as the entire cardiovascular system is devastated by rapidly constricting blood vessels. The sudden increase of blood pressure and heart rate after several deep inhalations of the freebase smoke can trigger convulsions and coronary attacks. Freebasing is known to repress several enzymes crucial to heart function.

Physical symptoms which commonly follow the abrupt cessation of chronic high-dose use include nausea, tremors, acute depression, irregular appetite and sleep patterns, anhedonia (inability to enjoy), intense drug craving, paranoia, and a schizophrenic psychosis. Hoarseness, bronchitis, and bloody expectorant are also reported by freebase smokers.

Dr. Sidney Schnoll of Northwestern University is doing research involving the organic and synthetic byproducts from freebase cocaine as well as the cocaine residues themselves that appear to be causing lung disease in users.

Residue is clearly visible on freebase paraphernalia such as bowls and stems of pipes, where recrystallization takes place during use. It is common practice to clean freebase equipment of residue with a strong solvent. A similar procedure cannot be done for the lungs.

Long-term effects of freebase are thought to cause permanent pulmonary damage as byproducts are deposited in the alveoli (air cells of the lungs), producing a significant reduction of carbon monoxide-diffusing capacity. This might be experienced as shortness or gasping for breath and a painful ache in the lungs.

I had a $700-a-day habit when I quit. My friend took me down to USC Hospital . . . I'd always been basing with straight ammonia. Then you just wash and rinse your product clean. I thought I was getting purer base than with soda . . . I think maybe quitting I can clean out the build-up in my lungs. Someone told me freebase only stayed 24 hours in your system. What's this black shit in my lungs then?

Flower wholesaler
West Coast
May 1986

Lung disease, brain seizures, heart attacks, repeated convulsions, ventricular fibrillation, and a host of other toxic effects are increasingly linked to freebase cocaine. Pulmonary edema and congestion of the viscera (internal organs) are two abnormalities found at autopsies of known freebasers that suggest polydrug use, especially heroin.

Freebasers sometimes take alcohol, sedatives, or narcotics such as heroin to come down off a binge that has made them hypertensive, paranoid, and unable to sleep. The notion that heroin may neutralize the effects of cocaine is dangerously untrue. Combined doses of cocaine and various narcotics depress the respiratory center. In a study of major cities in the United States, one-quarter of the cocaine-related deaths reveal the presence of narcotics.

Compelling evidence confirms that cocaine worsens pre-existing heart weaknesses and causes heart attacks. If a person suffers from even mild heart disease, the racing pulse and pounding heart that is set off by cocaine can lead to cardiac arrest.

Treatment

Access to a strong, viable peer group, such as Alcoholics Anonymous, Narcotics Anonymous, and Cocaine Anonymous, continues to be the most effective treatment.

"Personally, I advocate self-detoxification. Screw all these do-gooders."

Former speedfreak
New York City
July 1986

In South America they are doing brain surgery on adolescent cocaine users because they won't stop any other way, so they are going to cut out their pleasure centers. In our last WHO meetings in Bogota, they were pleased to report to us that 50% of the patients that they operated on stayed away from cocaine for a couple of months. Real nice. Irreversible procedure called a bilateral cingulotomy—something like the frontal lobotomies we used to practice in this country.

Dr. Ronald Siegel
Designer Drug Conference, UCLA
October 1985

Inside the Brain

Dr. Forrest Tennant, executive director of a network of general medical care clinics and drug treatment centers, addressed a group of narcotics officers taking his class on the neurochemistry of drug addiction at the California Narcotics Officers' 1985 Convention:

> Parents are riled. And I mean *riled.* I've never seen anything like it before. All of the sudden this drug problem has become unimaginable and they are scared. And they're doing something about it. They are learning about the drugs. They know what happens inside the brain. They are speaking in medical terms at their civic meetings. They have finally come to realize that *they* have to do something about this problem because law enforcement can't do it alone. And if you've got parents out there talking about damaged neurotransmitters and dopamine depletion—you'd better know what the hell they're talking about.

Freebasing cocaine disrupts the normal balance of three essential neurotransmitters (signal-carrying chemicals that broadcast messages within the body's nerve network): norepinephrine, serotonin, and dopamine.

Normally, norepinephrine (and possibly dopamine) is responsible for an individual's alertness, energy, and assertiveness. Its general purpose is to prep the body for immediate danger and emergency. Sudden release of norepinephrine mobilizes an individual for flight, aggression, or defense. Smoking freebase cocaine greatly increases norepinephrine neurotransmission, producing increased heart rate, dilation of the pupils, higher blood pressure, constriction of blood vessels in the skin and mucous membranes, increased blood sugar, rise in body temperature, and so on. At acute levels, behavior becomes extremely anxious, aggressive, and violent. Continued intense levels of stimulation may lead to death from cardiac arrest and respiratory failure.

Normally, the body uses its neurotransmitters, then reabsorbs them for future use. Cocaine, however, blocks that reabsorption, creating a shortage in the body. After the effects of cocaine wear off, a shortage of norepinephrine results in acute depression, lethargy, loss of appetite and sexual drive, and chronic fatigue.

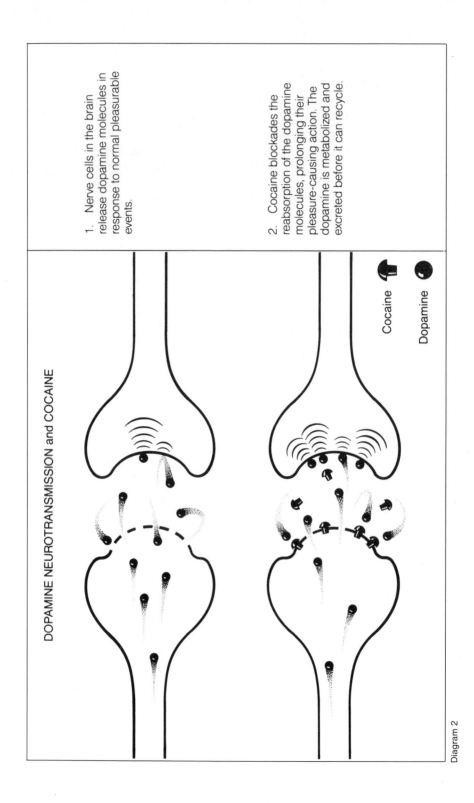

DOPAMINE NEUROTRANSMISSION and COCAINE

1. Nerve cells in the brain release dopamine molecules in response to normal pleasurable events.

2. Cocaine blockades the reabsorption of the dopamine molecules, prolonging their pleasure-causing action. The dopamine is metabolized and excreted before it can recycle.

Cocaine

Dopamine

Diagram 2

Freebased cocaine appears to depress neurotransmission of serotonin, which is responsible for the regulation of sleep. Insomnia and hyperactivity are the common symptoms. Jitteriness, paranoia, and insomnia invite multiple dependency in the form of alcohol, marijuana, sedatives, and heroin (which has been mentioned in Chapter 1 as a drug becoming more popular to smoke, not inject).

> It's funny but the guy who introduced me to it, who had a $2,000 habit, was with us out in California for the first time and when he was basing and showing us and getting high, he kept going over to the curtains and pulling them like a sixteenth of an inch closer together like someone was out on the street watching him who knew he'd just driven in from Ohio! Really paranoid! I wondered about that. Why get high if you're so incredibly paranoid. And he kept yelling at us about being careful we didn't tip over the bunsen burner!
>
> Electrician/musician
> San Fernando Valley, California
> May 1986

Dopamine, another neurotransmitter, is thought to be responsible for what individuals experience as euphoria and pleasure. Cells in the brain discharge dopamine into synapses—gaps between cells that relay messages. The dopamine then attaches to receptors and a signal to stop transmission is conveyed. The dopamine is immediately reabsorbed for future use. Smoking freebased cocaine (as well as snorting or shooting cocaine), however, blocks the reabsorption as it does with norepinephrine, causing prolonged activity in the synapses (see diagram 2). The effect is exhilaration. A feeling of superior confidence, power, and joyous excitement grips the user.

> I have no idea [how they smoke it]—I don't hang out with those people. I don't like being around people when they're on cocaine. When they're doing cocaine, you know what it's like, they get all pushy and rappy and didactic, jubilant, euphoric for no good reason. Screw that. I'll go sit in another room 'til you guys are through.
>
> Dean Latimer
> New York City
> November 1985

> I don't know if you call them coke whores. I mean a lot of
> these girls are nice girls. Just a little dumb . . . I'd always try
> and have sex with them *before* they got high because after-
> wards, what a waste . . . One thing I can't stand is endless
> chattering—pontificating and philosophizing about absolutely
> nothing. I mean they are hardly equipped to philosophize.
> We're talking bleak. Some of them drive me f—ing nuts!
> That's usually [when we are] snorting coke. Turn them onto
> freebase and you might as well be at the morgue.
>
> Businessman
> Former freebaser/dealer
> July 1986

The available dopamine supply is depleted, just as the norepinephrine supply is depleted, after frequent smoking of freebased cocaine.
As the acute effects of the drug wear off, the user craves more
cocaine. The user's uncontrollable craving for more cocaine has been
directly linked to the shortage of dopamine. For example, when an
artificial promoter of dopamine activity is prescribed, such as the
drug bromocriptine, the user's craving temporarily subsides. Imipramine is another drug working much the same way. The drugs bind
to the same sites in the brain that cocaine binds to and block its
action.

After each freebase binge, the body's supply of dopamine is
further depleted. Dr. Mark Gold suggested in his research paper,
"New Concepts in Cocaine Addiction: The Dopamine Depletion
Hypothesis," that the brain increases brain receptor sensitivity to
dopamine to make up for that depletion: "Increased receptor
sensitivity to compensate for DA (dopamine) deficiency would
amplify the effects of subsequent doses of cocaine. Thus, due to the
nature of neurotransmitter disruptions in cocaine use, tolerance
would not be expected." In short, Gold says sensitivity prevents
tolerance.

In other words, the receptors that receive the dopamine stimulus
become supersensitive to make up for the loss of some of the body's
dopamine supply. The receptors give the remaining dopamine
neurotransmitters a bigger chance to score with their receptors. That
would mean that when an artificial stimulant such as cocaine was
again used, the user would experience as strong an effect as

previously experienced and would not develop tolerance to the cocaine. Why, then, do cocaine freebasers feel compelled to up their dose, consuming larger and larger amounts?

You can do enough freebase to kill you and not realize it because the base numbs your lungs and you can keep sucking it in. After that first hit, you spend the rest of the night trying for that same rush. You keep hoping the next hit will do it, and you add more to the pipe and breathe in deeper, but it's never the same and I mean *never* the same. Nothing compares to that first hit.

Commercial illustrator
West Coast
July 1986

Freebasers always talk about their first time and how their consumption of the drug steadily increases. The compulsion then to up the dose appears to be a question not of tolerance to the drug but, rather, of users chasing an elusive high which may never again be repeated because users may never have that great a supply of neurotransmitters again. Thus, the first time users freebase, the cocaine freebase activates more neurotransmitters than will ever be possible again. No matter how hard the brain tries to compensate for that lost supply of neurotransmitters (which the body metabolizes and excretes), no matter how hard the brain tries to make up that loss through increased sensitivity, the user's first explosive rush of euphoria will never be felt again.

With chronic freebasing, the body's natural supply of dopamine continues to be depleted. The dopamine is metabolized and excreted before the body can reabsorb it and replenish its limited supply. The user's ability to experience pleasure and euphoria is dramatically altered. The simplest pleasures like an afternoon nap, a soothing melody, a breath of fresh air, the warm touch of a friend seem oddly empty of joy. The body's natural chemical mechanism for making the person feel good has been damaged. The user has been self-conditioned to seek an outside artificial stimulus to replace that lost joy. The user craves more cocaine.

Some researchers believe that chronic use of concentrated forms of cocaine like Crack and Rock may cause a *permanent* depletion of certain neurotransmitters as well as cause irreparable damage to brain receptors. One researcher likens damaged brain receptors to "dented car fenders" (injured by the sudden onslaught of neurotransmitters triggered by extremely potent freebased cocaine). The implications for recovery are unsettling.

As mentioned above, commercially available prescription drugs, such as bromocriptine and imipramine, work to temporarily relieve the drug-craving in chronic users. But the drugs are only a temporary replacement for cocaine. A crucial question being raised by researchers is whether or not the body can naturally regenerate neurotransmitters, synthesizing a new supply to replace those lost from cocaine use. Giving the user supplementary vitamins that would supply the basic precursors needed by the body to synthesize new neurotransmitters has been talked about but not yet researched.

I am not aware of any published studies that confirm the permanent depletion theory. We think the normal building blocks are there to help eventually restore the body's depleted neurotransmitters.

Dr. Carter Pottash
Fair Oaks Hospital
Summit, New Jersey
June 1986

Irrespective of pharmacological interventions, psychological approaches at present remain the most important aspect of treatment for cocaine addiction . . . Self-help groups and education are quite effective in treating the vast majority of cocaine patients who are motivated for abstinence. The admission of powerlessness over cocaine is an important step for the addict, and a prerequisite to accepting outside help and direction.

Dr. Mark Gold
"New Concepts in Cocaine Addiction"
October 1984

I just bought this [a marble-size rock of freebase] from the taxi-driver. He says at least I didn't lose a house in Beverly Hills or a bunch of money. I haven't got anything so I got nothin' to lose. I don't say it to rationalize but it's true, I got nothin' to lose. I was just up at the psychic. She says I'm never gonna have kids.

I use 151 rum because it's the best, healthiest way [to ignite freebase]. Basing [street cocaine] yourself is dangerous cuz you never quit. This is the first time I've smoked in two years. I'm liking what Alcoholics Anonymous is saying, and I'm getting ready to quit a *lot* of drugs so I'm just doing this one last time.

Shooting coke—oh god—it's the best. I did it back in Tucson. I don't have hardly any scars left . . . When I was basing two years ago with my wife and doing it every night, it used to make me *so* sick! I'd puke all over the place.

My dealer has a theory about this Crack. He says they came up with that word cuz when basers smoke a long time sometimes their pipe will get so hot it'll crack. So Crack caught on as the "in" word for people into basing. Isn't this wild how rampant it is? I just can't believe that many people are doing it. Jesus.

What I'm doing I know is evil and wicked. It really is. I know that. Only two things worse are PCP and shooting up. I'm joining AA. What they're talking about in there is a lot of good things.

Gourmet chef
Los Angeles
July 1986

Freebase and the Unborn

Few studies have been conducted to test the effects of cocaine use on the unborn. Women who seek treatment for cocaine dependency while pregnant offer the rare opportunity to study such effects. A study published in the *New England Journal of Medicine* on September 12, 1985, involved twenty-three cocaine-using pregnant women. The women were divided into two groups. Group 1 had conceived while using cocaine and many continued using cocaine during the pregnancy. Group 2 conceived while using cocaine and heroin. They were given methadone as a replacement for the heroin during the pregnancy, but many continued using cocaine. Both groups were compared to women who used narcotics only in the past and were maintained on methadone during the pregnancy (Group 3); Group 4 consisted of drug-free pregnant women.

During the pregnancies, four of the cocaine-using women went into labor prematurely and experienced detachment of the placenta after injecting a single dose of cocaine (effects of freebasing cocaine have been equated with intravenous use of cocaine).

Additionally, one infant of a cocaine-using mother was born with malformations of the genitourinary tract. A second infant died of meningitis and a third infant died of Sudden Infant Death Syndrome. Groups 3 and 4 had none of the above problems.

Babies whose mothers used cocaine while pregnant have been born with congenital abnormalities, according to Dr. Judy Howard, medical director of UCLA's Suspected Child Abuse and Neglect Team. Chromosomal defects such as ears placed too low or eyes set too far apart developed during the pregnancy. At birth, some babies have appeared catatonic after suffering numerous small strokes caused by abrupt changes in the mother's blood pressure.

A baby in the Midwest was born half-paralyzed from a stroke—a stroke that occurred as a result of the mother binging on cocaine during her pregnancy.

Dr. Michael Weitzman, director of maternal health at Boston City Hospital in Massachusetts, said that two women, thirty-four weeks pregnant, went into labor that was more intense than normal after using cocaine. Heart rates of both fetuses dropped in half, possibly reducing oxygen to the brain. Doctors were forced to deliver the babies prematurely by emergency Caesarean section to prevent brain damage and death.

More and more studies are leading researchers to believe that cocaine causes spontaneous abortion and premature detachment of the placenta and that infants exposed to cocaine during pregnancy have a higher rate of neurologic behavior problems, congenital malformations, and death.

The Law

Crack is a form of cocaine which is a Schedule II drug: high abuse potential with restricted medical use. Statutes vary considerably from state to state with a wide range of penalties: ninety days to twenty years for first conviction for possession and stiffer sentences for the sale of cocaine.

Synthetic Cocaine

Synthetic cocaine is prohibitive to cook up on the black market because it is expensive and time consuming. Dozens of other low-yield recipes for synthetic cocaine circulate on the black market. In most cases, synthetic tropacocaine—one of the alkaloids in coca which is related to cocaine—is produced. Tropacocaine commonly triggers belladonna-like effects including hallucinations, dizziness, fever, confusion, rapid pulse and breathing, slurred speech, convulsions and coma.

[During the] mid-70s, cocaine got big very fast. I toyed with the idea of synthesizing it. Nobody knew anything about the process. I took time off to research it and spent several months in Germany and then on the East Coast. It took a long time to get a decent enough lab yield. One major obstacle was duplicating the physical properties of cocaine. I worked with maybe six different analogs, mixing and matching, until I had identical stereochemical aspects. With liquid chromatography, I cleaned up the impurities and was ready to do business. I sold it as rocked up crystal cocaine. That is quite an accomplishment. I don't know anybody that has done it since— which isn't to say there aren't a bunch out there trying. The research was really indispensable . . . I was only in the business a short time as it got to be very, very dangerous. Nobody in the coke trade can be trusted. Not the people working for you—I was repeatedly ripped off—not your suppliers, not the dealers, nobody. And everyone packs a gun. I was constantly breaking down and relocating my lab. The major conflict was, of course, territorial. When you're turning out LSD, PCP, methamphetamine—that sort of thing—you more often than not do business with dealer-users on the street. But with lumps of synthetic rock cocaine, you undercut organized crime distributors and you are in big trouble. You don't want to mess with those fellows, I don't care how much money you're making. I quit the business to save my neck.

Convicted PCP chemist
West Coast penitentiary
September 1985

"As with any other molecule, cocaine can be modified in the
lab to make it more potent," warns Frank Sapienza . . . By
means of a difficult and expensive process, U.S. scientists have
successfully synthesized cocaine, and drug-enforcement officials
expect private suppliers could make it as well if natural cocaine
ever becomes scarce.

U.S. News and World Report
July 28, 1986

The state of California recently passed legislation placing all
synthetic cocaine analogs, salt isomers, and preparations thereof in
the same classification as natural cocaine, mandating identical
penalties and fines for possession or sales. This was done in response
to criminal cases in which authorities were unable to distinguish
natural from synthetic cocaine without a device called a polarimeter.

Cocaine . . . has been designer produced to create the freebase
phenomenon which is responsible for the rapid proliferation of
cocaine abuse in our society. It affects every segment of our
society today. I'm everywhere—I'm over at the big industry
corporations, I'm with professional sports teams, I'm with
playgrounds—eight-year-old kids in grammar school in San
Francisco . . . It's permeated every level of our society, no
matter how you want to measure it.

For example, I was on "Live On 4" in San Francisco a couple
years ago and they had asked me on to talk about the cocaine
epidemic in San Francisco . . . At the same time I was on that
show there was also a DEA agent on that show. This Drug
Enforcement [agent] interrupts me during my rap and says,
"Doctor Inaba, that might be true but the DEA is not going
to allow this situation to get out of hand. We're going to be
able to control the cocaine coming into America."

Now when I had walked into the studio, he had sitting right
next to him a German Shepherd and I thought he might be
sight-impaired or something. So now he points down to this
German Shepherd and he says, "We have just trained a
hundred of these dogs right here. These dogs can sniff out a
tenth of a milligram of cocaine no matter where anybody tries

to conceal it. These dogs became famous last year—they sniffed out 2 tons of cocaine coming into New York in refrigerators . . .''

So he's saying these dogs are so effective that he—as the studio audience members were filing in—he slipped a bindle, a little package folded up containing a tenth of a milligram of cocaine, and he asked one of the studio audience members to hold it as he's going to let this dog go, and the dog will find it in a second.

Now I'm sitting there looking at the talk show host and his eyes get *real* wide and he's getting real scared and I'm thinking—My God, what's going on here?! I just told him cocaine was everywhere. We're in San Francisco—dope capital of the world. We're in a TV station . . . and I do a lot of employee assistance work with TV media people because cocaine's rampant there. We're thinking, boy, there's gonna be mass confusion! He lets the dog go, and the dog goes straight for the drummer. One of the most amazing things I've ever seen. Straight for the drummer, and the drummer stands up and says, ''Excuse me''—we're live on TV—and he goes to the bathroom and the DEA agent is looking perplexed. The talk show host and I start talking about the cocaine harvest—the boom crop in South America and the guy is still saying, ''But it should've been over with this guy here . . .''

We don't know if he ever caught on, but the situation is cocaine has permeated every level of our society and what we're seeing is designer cocaine in the form of rock cocaine which is the based cocaine (using) baking soda and a torch. Shake it and heat it. Shake it and heat it. The thing congeals into a rock and you put that rock right into a pipe, heat it up . . . and inhale it.

Dr. Darryl Inaba
Designer Drug Conference, UCLA
October 1985

Doonesbury

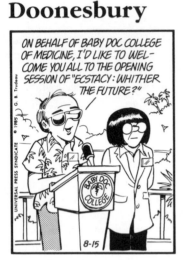

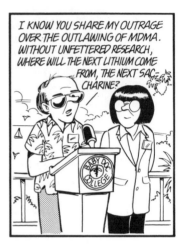

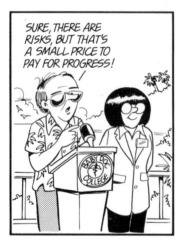

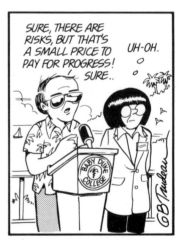

4 "Ecstasy"

◆ *You should go into your first Ecstasy sharing with the understanding that you are going to have a beautiful, relaxed experience, that your heart is going to open totally to feelings of love, that you will not have any anxiety actions, that you will alter your consciousness in such a way that when the experience is over you will take something from the experience that will enrich your life, and that you can expect to have virtually no physical sensations that will in any way impair you or make you feel uncomfortable. You will have no aftereffects such as a hangover type of feeling, or a buzz in your head the next day. In fact, the day after Ecstasy is perhaps even more pleasant than the actual experience because you feel like you are floating like a butterfly the whole day, and yet you are very much in tune with what you are doing and the work that you are doing that day compared to your average workaday world, because you are more in tune with your body, your mind, and your senses.*

Ecstasy: 21st Century Entheogen
(Underground pamphlet distributed by
marketers of MDMA)

Million Dollar Baby

In late 1984 and early 1985, word of a new magical elixir swept the country promising to assuage life's emotional ills. It could mend marriages, cure alcohol and cocaine addiction, help the dying face death, console rape victims, remove writer's block, and allow thousands of self-serving yuppies to empathize.

What was this twenty-first-century nepenthe? This new "hug drug" to promote world peace through blissed-out intimacy? This drug worthy enough to be tested by the government as a potential agent to turn hostile civilians into purring pussycats?

Ecstasy! a.k.a. "XTC" a.k.a. "Adam" and also known as MDMA to researchers, the medical community, and a group of black-market chemists and users familiar with the drug from the 1960s. Originally synthesized in the early 1900s, MDMA is considered the licit parent (and illicit daughter) of MDA (the "love drug") and methamphetamine ("speed").

It was a drug considered for use as an appetite suppressant but never manufactured because it gave you the heaves. A drug surfacing, then disappearing during the 1960s counterculture because LSD-25 was delivering ten times the punch and you didn't have to get sick to enjoy it. A drug popular among psychotherapists during the 1970s and 1980s because it was remarkably similar to LSD-25 in small doses and was, most importantly, legal. A drug that a handful of clever California entrepreneurs decided to resurrect, christen, package, market, distribute, and advertise. A marketing million dollar baby. Ecstasy.

Interview: Large man. Late thirties. Well-known stage and television actor.

I do Ecstasy twice a month. I take two hits in the space of eight hours. For example, I'll take one at 4 P.M. Saturday and then one at 8 P.M. Taking two or three over the course of Saturday P.M. to Sunday A.M. can be dehydrating, so I take minerals and vitamins during that time despite a lack of appetite. The residual effect is debilitating—not unlike the lag after a coke run, so the minerals and vitamins are important.

There are various realms of abstraction which depend heavily on the individual. I never hallucinate. Some of my friends do. The more far out the artist or the creative, the more pronounced the hallucinogenic effect. It goes with the territory. A certain intensity in the experience gives the illusion of substance to the alter ego. Gary Trudeau captured that in his "Doonesbury" cartoons. I find it to be incredibly true.

Generally speaking, there is a fundamental good feeling. It's fun. There is an empathy. A calmer understanding. You feel kind and loving. An aphrodisiac, very sensual feeling.

I first started taking Ecstasy five years ago with one other person. Today, there are four or five of us who consistently use it. Those are the only people I personally know about. Word of mouth is that the big buys are for the movie and record people.

Different personalities react differently. The "controlled" type of guy always throws up. If you resist, you'll throw it up. You see a lot of tensing. A lot of grinding teeth. Some can't get to sleep. I can. The high lasts four to five hours. The availability is there. Price keeps me from buying now. After its scheduling, it shot up in price. I was paying $8 to $25. Now it's up over $30. That makes a pretty expensive evening. The people I know don't abuse it. When the price goes up, they refrain. It's just not that important. Of course, there will always be the group who abuses—be it food, alcohol, or drugs. Just because they are greedy and irresponsible, why take it away from the rest of us?

I know nothing about quality control, I have no idea how many milligrams I'm taking. I trust a friend. I don't ask questions. I know it comes from Texas.

Los Angeles
November 1985

Interview: Woman in her late thirties. Creative director in fashion advertising.

I've been taking Ecstasy probably ten years. I buy directly from a lab which relocated mid-1985. It's pharmaceutical Ecstasy and I sell it uncut. I sell it for what I pay for it. I'm not dealing. Just a connection for good friends. I always send cash. Usually $1,000 or more. Always through the mail.

"X" makes me feel like I'm twelve years old again. That's the best description I can give. A gentle, innocent state of mind. A week's worth of stress at work, problems at home with bills, the kids, even the marriage suddenly aren't taken so seriously. Life becomes simple again.

On the average, I'd take it every three weeks. I can't really do it more often because I'm exhausted for three days after each experience. The only bad experience I know about happened to a friend of mine. It was the first time she took it and she was sicker than a dog all night. I should have told her to take half a tab.

Recently, since I've been divorced, I haven't used it in a number of weeks. I've cut down mainly because my new boyfriend would rather I didn't do any drugs at all. That's one of the nice things about Ecstasy. You can quit without any regrets. Would I recommend it to my kids? I don't want my kids doing *any* drugs. Mature responsible adults can decide for themselves. Not kids. The stuff's too easy to abuse.

Los Angeles
April 1986

Nothing New

In 1576, Lobelius in his *Plantarum Seu Stiripium Historia* recorded for the first time nutmeg's hallucinogenic effects on a "pregnant English lady who, having eaten ten or twelve nutmegs, became deliriously inebriated." (Nutmeg may have at that time undeservedly earned the reputation of being an abortifacient.) In 1829, Purkinje, a famous biologist, ate three nutmegs and found the euphoria strikingly similar to Cannabis (marijuana) intoxication. A similar insight was later shared by Malcolm X while in prison. In his autobiography, he tells of dumping a matchbox full of nutmeg into a glass of water and drinking it—the equivalent (for Mr. X) of smoking four reefers. Freshly grated nutmeg will produce a profound intoxication and a variety of visual, auditory, and tactile hallucinations depending on the individual.

I got two hits. A gift from my son. He's been dealing Ecstasy. We're having some problems with him. But, uh, I mostly remember my jaws were wired shut. Not my idea of a great high. My favorite drug of all time is DMT—dimethyltryptamine. Imagine standing 100 yards away from a tree and seeing the leaves as if they were inches away—every living vivid detail and the rushing freight train sound of them shaking in the wind!

Writer/actor
Hollywood, California
March 1986

I hallucinated. I didn't know Ecstasy made you hallucinate.
Little people up on the bookshelf. And my jaws felt wired shut
too. All night long. I kept wondering when do I get to make
love? His son apologized. Said it was cut with speed. He didn't
realize I don't do a lot of drugs.

Girlfriend of writer/actor
Hollywood, California
March 1986

A person under the spell of nutmeg is likely to find himself
unable actually to sleep, but also incapable of being really
awake. Sleepless stupor is the most apt description of nutmeg
narcosis . . . The aftereffects are usually quite unpleasant:
aching of the bones and muscles, soreness and aching of the
eyes, running nose, tiredness, depression and possible headaches. One of the best things that can be said about nutmeg
intoxication is that it is too unpleasant to be addicting.

The First Book Of Sacraments
of the Church of the Tree of Life

Whether derived from the oils of nutmeg, sassafras, mace, saffron,
calamus, crocus, or parsley, or synthesized in a laboratory, MDMA
is a psychoactive drug with hallucinogenic and amphetaminergic
properties. Its chemical structure, 3,4 methylenedioxy-methamphe-
tamine, is molecularly related to nutmeg and two synthetic drugs,
MDA and methamphetamine. It is chemically similar to mescaline
and the nasal decongestant Sudafed (Pseudoephedrine).

Gays are doing a lot of crystal and now and then a little
MDMA. You'll bust one with so much methamphetamine and
maybe a little MDMA. When they do them together, they
aren't prepared for the combined stimulant and hallucinogen
and sometimes it freaks them out.

Narcotics detective
West Hollywood, California
December 1985

In 1914, E. Merck, a German pharmaceutical firm, synthesized
MDMA as a possible appetite suppressant. It was never manufactured because of the drug's potential physical liabilities.

Even the people who have unlimited supplies of it, the distributors and the traffickers, are afraid to take a lot of it to test the limits. We do have some brave explorers that always will go way out there. They have a hard time articulating because I've found that there's a continuing problem with speech in these people that seems to persist for a long period of time . . . They have muscular difficulties, coordination difficulties, especially in speech. I'm talking about pushing the dose up to 300, 400, 500 milligrams . . . But let's say 135 is being used . . . we're looking at some very toxic effects. We're looking at nausea, vomiting—that's a message from the alkaloids that are starting to poison you while it's turning you on. Most drugs will give you an altered experience, an altered state of consciousness just before they poison you—that's part of the trip.

Dr. Ronald Siegel
Designer Drug Conference, UCLA
October 1985

Underground literature on MDMA claims that Alexander Shulgin was the scientist who invented Ecstasy; that he was paid by the CIA to develop the ultimate truth serum; and that Ecstasy was his contribution. Shulgin, in fact, is a specialist working in areas related to mescaline and is credited as the initial synthesizer of STP and MMDA. In 1962, Shulgin first recorded the effects of MMDA and has written extensively on the subject.

In 1953, the U.S. Army covertly tested MDMA, code name EA-1475, as an "experimental agent" at its Edgewood arsenal in Maryland. Although never tested in man, it was found to be highly toxic to monkeys and dogs, causing convulsions and death in large doses. It was declassified in 1967, and first published in the scientific literature in 1973.

The DEA first identified MDMA in the illicit drug traffic in 1970. A number of black-market chemists had synthesized it during the 1960s but found LSD and MDA to be more profitable. Because there was little street abuse of the drug, it was not scheduled by the federal government.

In the mid-1970s a group of entrepreneurs/chemists decided to set up a lab in Marin County, California, to manufacture MDMA. Marketing ideas and a variety of salable names were discussed.

"Empathy" was seriously considered, as the drug seemed to elicit a user's more compassionate nature. "Ecstasy" was selected for having a bit more pizzazz.

> Our friends do it on the weekends. They feel very special and think nobody can tell they are high. Bullshit. They glide around like Mr. and Mrs. Perfect, real quiet, real mellow. So when you go out to eat or have them over for dinner you don't have to worry if there's going to be enough food to go around because they're never hungry! Also, if you're short cash for the movies, you can ask 'em for the extra bucks and they'll never remember loaning it to you!
>
> Female, late twenties
> Lake Arrowhead, California
> January 1986

The lab operated for five years before relocating. The drug was marketed with package inserts, some of which included unverified scientific research and an abundance of 1960s mumbo-jumbo.

> All Ecstasy does is open the doors to your higher self, and sometimes, people don't like what they see. Even though they have a beautiful first experience with Ecstasy, the next day they say, "Well that wasn't the real me!" and they totally invalidate the beautiful experience they had because it is not something that they are familiar with, or comfortable with, or willing to deal with . . . The greatest benefit of Ecstasy is the clarity of vision you have about yourself, and that clarity comes with enough psychic energy to make the necessary changes for increased health and loving relationships in your life.
>
> *Ecstasy: 21st Century Entheogen*

Surprisingly good advice on the "safe" use of the drug was given, including an adamant warning against using it in combination with other drugs or alcohol, using the drug sparingly over an extended period of time, and being extremely cautious about the environment and the people with whom the drug is taken—guidance not unlike that which the Indians offered their own people when using peyote for ceremonial consumption.

> Don't eat for at least eight hours . . . drink only pure distilled
> or mineral water. Do not mix it with alcohol or any drugs
> (such as marijuana, cocaine or downers), or anything else . . .
> The best experience for Ecstasy results from when you save
> them for special occasions and the right circumstances and the
> right people . . . taking it to get yourself out of bad moods
> only intensifies those moods . . . If you take it with someone
> you feel uncomfortable with, it may intensify that discomfort
> to an unbearable degree. Therefore, when you do Ecstasy,
> please be extremely careful about when, where and with whom
> you do it.
>
> *Ecstasy: 21st Century Entheogen*

In 1976, the lab known to be producing MDMA was distributing approximately 10,000 doses per month throughout the United States. By 1984, the same lab had escalated production to 30,000 doses. By mid-1985, a combined distribution among the flourishing number of distributors was estimated to be nearly a half-million doses per month. At that time, the drug was available in at least twenty-one states and Canada. Areas of concentration were California, Texas, Florida, New York, and New England. Distribution was said to have reached Portugal and Spain and parts of South America.

News stories in *Newsweek* (April 1985), *New York Magazine* (May 1985), *Time* (June 1985), and *Life* (August 1985) published claims about MDMA's psychotherapeutic benefits. A sudden demand for the drug for which there was no supply was met instead by street hustlers eager to cash in on the trend. PCP was sold in Chicago as Ecstasy. MDA was sold in New York as Ecstasy. Elsewhere throughout the country, a variety of other drugs were misrepresented as Ecstasy, including caffeine, LSD, ephedrine, and DOM.

> After the article in *New York* was published we were getting
> calls on our Hotline from people wanting to know where they
> could buy "Ecstasy"!
>
> Dr. Mark Gold
> Fair Oaks Hospital
> Summit, New Jersey
> November 1985

Why sell LSD as MDMA when the LSD's a quality product? We confiscated just last month 60,000 hits of 4-way Mickey Mouse acid. We were buying sheets [that] broken down were maybe 37 cents a hit. 60% purity. Excellent LSD. Bunch of Grateful Dead freaks had it made for their own little group. Paper blotter lab. One guy. No phone. Out in the boonies. Never, never catch him. Who wants MDMA?

State narcotics agent
San Francisco, California
October 1985

When MDMA became very popular we had a lot of samples in the Haight [Ashbury District] of MDA—chemists who had MDA available were calling their stuff "Adam" and "Ecstasy" and we analyzed them and maybe that's how MDMA got the rap where there were three deaths involved with it. Those really have to be questioned because it seems like maybe those deaths might have been due to MDA instead of MDMA.

Dr. Darryl Inaba
Designer Drug Conference, UCLA
October 1985

It was during this period of Ecstacy frenzy that an estimated 500 MDMA-related crises were reported at emergency rooms and drug abuse clinics involving severe anxiety reactions, paranoia, depression, and a few well-publicized psychotic episodes and deaths.

Delusional, paranoid, rapid heartbeat, prolonged depression . . . these people had taken 5 to 15 hits of MDMA.

Dr. Darryl Inaba
Designer Drug Conference, UCLA
October 1985

We've dropped three to five doses at a time either eating or whiffing our last dose when we start coming down. It's like levels [climbing stairs] taking three to four doses at once. Just when you think you've peaked, you peak again, then again— each hit a "peak"—three hits equaling three "peaks," get it? Anyway, after two peaks [doses], we all agree it starts getting intense, not like a calm Ecstasy trip, more like a horror movie.

"Users Speak Out"
High Times
November 1985

I only heard about one bad case with MDMA. The only
reason I heard about it, some guy called up here [*High Times*]
saying he'd taken MDMA a couple weeks before and now his
vision was a little weird. I recommended him to the Haight-
Ashbury Free Clinic. They're great people. I got treated for
clap by the Haight Clinic first year it was in existence. I was a
hippie in 1966.

> Reporter
> *High Times*
> November 1985

I have never seen a case from an MDMA type of drug and I
include MDA or nutmeg or anything like that—I have never
seen a case come in for clinical treatment.

> Dr. Ronald Siegel
> Designer Drug Conference, UCLA
> October 1985

By July 1, 1985, the DEA had placed MDMA into Schedule I of
the Controlled Substances Act alongside heroin, LSD, MDA,
marijuana and other drugs considered to have high potentials for
abuse, no accepted medical use, and no safety standards accepted by
the Food and Drug Administration. The emergency measures made
trafficking in MDMA punishable by fifteen years in prison and a
$125,000 fine; and possession, a misdemeanor punishable by up to
five years in prison.

One of the things we have to advise users about is the legal
risks. They are very dangerous to your health. Getting caught.
As far as contamination and could you get Parkinson's disease
from MDMA—I don't know of any cases. And even if there
were, that isn't going to be the probability. Probability is that
you'll get busted and someone will make an example of you
because they want to come down on MDMA.

> Dr. Ronald Siegel
> Designer Drug Conference, UCLA
> October 1985

What's on the Street

After the scheduling, several distributors withdrew from the market. Labs were shut down by the DEA in Texas and Florida. One lab was intercepted on its way to Mexico. According to underground sources, the major distributors relocated and the original distribution network operating since the 1970s continues supplying the "Consciousness Circle" of users: users in their thirties, experienced with psychedelics, and not prone to abuse of the drugs.

Precursor for MDMA is isosafrol, which is also used for MDA. In Texas, we'd been watching for years and years the sale of isosafrol for MDA production. It is highly unlikely that manufacturers stockpiled isosafrol without DEA knowledge. They may possibly be making the isosafrol.

> DEA group head
> Clandestine Labs
> West Coast
> October 1985

There's still one major lab that produces Ecstasy . . . There was a lot of stockpiling of the precursor chemicals because one of the strategies now in the Administration's war on drugs is to try and proscribe the precursor chemicals . . . The chemicals that are necessary to make MDMA have been gathered up from around the world and stockpiled. There's a two-year supply available now to this laboratory. So for the next two years, they'll be able to handle production without any interference from any legislative controls.

> Dr. Ronald Siegel
> Designer Drug Conference, UCLA
> October 1985

After the scheduling, the price of Ecstasy shot up and the purer forms of the drug became scarce. Price increased from an average of $100 per gram to $300 per gram.

Black-market entrepreneurs continued selling adulterated versions or misrepresenting altogether different drugs.

> The worst and second most popular form is powder form—
> either white or yellow-brown with a lot of cut. Usually the
> dealer will get pure white Ecstasy [ten doses in a gram] and
> add about a third of a gram of procaine to give a strong
> nummie effect [one dealer told me it's supposed to get the coke
> addict hooked]. Anyway, after they're done stepping on it,
> they have about 1.3 grams of shit, which they cut into 1-12
> doses which will probably get your kid sister or a dwarf off,
> but for the everyday drug taker you'll have to take two doses
> to get off.
>
> "Users Speak Out"
> *High Times*
> October 1985

Street names for MDMA include "XTC," "Adam," "Ecstasy," "MDMA," and the "Love Drug." Initially, MDMA was sold with package inserts: "Ecstasy, Everything Looks Wonderful When You're Young and On Drugs," "Flight Instructions for a Friend Using XTC," "How to Prepare for an Ecstasy Experience," and "Ecstasy: 21st Century Entheogen."

Physical Properties, Adulterants

When purchased directly from the lab, it is a white powder in its purest form, tends to have a strong medicinal taste, and is often packaged in clear gelatin capsules. In that form it is rare and expensive, exceeding $35 a dose.

> We have a hard time confirming them [street samples] pharma-
> cologically because the price is so high. People don't want to
> part with the samples for analysis. The street price for MDMA
> is $30 in LA now. That is a yuppie drug! . . . You have to buy
> 500 to get the price down to $10. And that's still expensive.
>
> Dr. Ron Siegel
> Designer Drug Conference, UCLA
> October 1985

MDMA has been sold as a yellowish or white pill weighing one gram and nine-tenths cut with speed, caffeine, ephedrine, or other amphetamine cut. It has most recently been available as a white tab or pill. In April 1986, MDMA was selling at 100 hits for $350 in the Midwest (most probably adulterated). At the same time on the West Coast, adulterated versions were selling for $10 a dose and the quality MDMA for $20 or more. It is interesting that by April 1986 only three reports of MDMA were noted in *High Times,* compared to twenty-seven reports from across the country for LSD. Many of the drug seizures and samples tested at drug abuse clinics indicate that doses of MDMA on the street are low—as little as fifteen milligrams.

A friend just offered me ten hits at ten bucks apiece. I didn't buy it. I mean she's got a really good source but, you know, I just can't afford to be out of it even for two days. I've got too much work to do right now. I did some coke last night—two stinking lines and now I'm totally congested. Really pisses me off.

Graphic artist
Toluca Lake, California
February 1986

A segment of organized crime was said to have been approached by the California marketers of Ecstasy to act as distributors. The "bikers" are known to have a monopoly on the methamphetamine market throughout the country. The marketers of MDMA thought their drug could be plugged into this already established network. The bikers refused for three reasons: (1) MDMA is not addictive and cannot guarantee repetitive use; (2) users of the drug were too exclusive (not ubiquitous like speed and cocaine users); and (3) no big profit margin.

Effects on Users

At low doses, MDMA is mildly intoxicating, nonhallucinogenic, and has few physical liabilities. Toxic effects become noticeable at 100 to 200 milligrams. The following list of benefits and adverse effects is taken from the informed consent forms for people taking MDMA in psychotherapeutic sessions.

Potential Positive Effects

—enhanced alertness and mental clarity;

—more positive mood, feelings, and attitudes toward self and others;

—increased ability to effectively work on problems and conflicts in lives and relationships; and

—increased emotional warmth and love and greater ease in accepting both positive and negative expressions.

The XTC drugs are not genital aphrodisiacs. The extraordinary sensuality of the experience is generalized over the body. At the height of the session, caressing is the standard mode of communication, and after 3 or 4 hours, sexual relations may be in order.

Dr. Timothy Leary
Chic Magazine

Potential Adverse Effects

—muscle tightness;

—involuntary teeth-clenching and biting inside of cheek (relieved by placing damp washcloth between teeth and cheek);

—nausea with or without vomiting;

—dehydration;

—muscle aches and pains (can persist for six weeks);

—restlessness;

—shaking in the jaw;

—eyes become dry enough to cause swelling around eyes and blurred vision;

—intermittent rapid eye movement;

—decreased sensitivity to physical pain (care should be taken with chewing or swallowing or any vomiting in case debris goes down your windpipe);

—pulse and blood pressure fluctuation;

—sugar level fluctuation; and

—occasional visual hallucinations with geometric patterns, trails of moving objects.

I will relate to you an experience that I had when I tested a dose of Ecstasy that was thirty times the recommended amount. I had profuse sweating, body tremors, sensory changes such as blurred vision, multiple imagery, vibration of objects, increased passage of time and increased contrast . . . My psychic phenomenon was the loss of thought control, extreme elation, difficulty in expressing myself precisely, floods of thought or blankness of mind and ease of distraction. At no time during the overdose period was I alarmed or panicked, and my wife was never concerned enough to ask me would I like to go to the hospital.

Ecstasy: 21st Century Entheogen

I used to take it. My girlfriend does it every weekend and throws up every time. I prefer mushrooms. Psilocybin. I can function, I laugh, have a good time, and I know nobody's been messing with my stuff cuz I grow my own. I honestly don't know why she likes it.

Male fashion model
Los Angeles
December 1985

To me it felt like a very sophisticated, extremely well-buffered speed. You get the glow without the jitters (or the energy to write term papers). Once any discomfort has passed the only bad parts of the buzz are a mad passion for cigarettes and that grimy feeling on the skin common to many drugs . . . there have been claims that Ecstasy provides 'instant psychoanalysis' . . . Myself, I didn't come up with a unified field theory or anything. To really enjoy drugs, you've got to want to get out of where you are . . . But what drug will get a grownup out of, for instance, debt? . . . I slept fretfully, getting up every single hour to go to the bathroom. The next day the drug was still in my system. I felt okay but was a little disoriented, like I was in the next room and couldn't quite hear me . . . On the second day, all effects were gone, but I was tired and depressed."X" lag is pretty substantial for such a toy flip-out. A long run for a short slide. TUNE IN. TURN ON. GO TO THE OFFICE LATE ON MONDAY.

P.J. O'Rourke
Rolling Stone

MDMA is considered dangerous to anyone with a medical history of heart disease, diabetes, hypertension, epilepsy, hypoglycemia, glaucoma, psychotic episodes, or to anyone, as one doctor put it, "stupid enough to take multiple doses in their search for Nirvana."

Drowsiness and mild depression can accompany the delirium and last as long as three days.

MDMA vs Other Psychedelics

Dr. Ronald Siegel, psychopharmacologist at UCLA School of Medicine, has been conducting government-sponsored research on more than 170 MDMA users over an extended period of time. He is quoted at length throughout this chapter, his comments edited from a talk he gave at a conference on designer drugs held at UCLA in October 1985. He has also done extensive research on a variety of psychedelic drugs besides MDMA.

> I think that with mescaline where we have a lot of experience, we see that doses of 100 and 200 milligrams are virtually identical to the doses of MDMA on the street now. When we gave 400 and 800 milligrams of mescaline, we were getting so many physical complaints that the subjects were being distracted from the intensified mental effects and were preoccupied with the nausea and the vomiting. The nausea especially which just never went away and stayed for like 16 hours into the trip. Same thing happens with nutmeg. You increase the dose, you increase the physical effects as well as the mental effects.
>
> So the MDMA users have kept the dose real low, and by keeping the dose real low they think they have a unique drug—they don't. In fact, I can make an argument pharmacologically

that LSD and psilocybin are much safer than MDMA because we have a paucity of physical effects with LSD. We have a paucity of physical effects with psilocybin. Psilocybin is universally loved by everyone we gave it to and on the street, too. It's a very popular street psychedelic. You can grow your own. You know it's pure because the spores are sold through the mail and you can cultivate your own little mushroom garden. MDMA has a long recovery period. The effects are long. And it drains people.

Scheduling vs Research

A prestigious group of researchers, psychologists, psychiatrists, and lawyers demanded that MDMA be placed in the less restrictive Schedule III, which allows medical use and research. They argue that it should be left up to the medical profession and not the government to decide what is or is not accepted medical practice.

Experts from prestigious medical schools are again saying there is no proof of dangerousness [as they did for cocaine]. New medicines are normally assumed to be dangerous until proven safe and effective, but this policy, which has saved America from hundreds of Thalidomides, is lost when it comes to drugs of abuse. New drugs are peculiarly exempt from medical logic and viewed as safe until proven dangerous . . . MDA, MDMA and MMDA should be viewed on the basis of studies with similar drugs and research work with these drugs in animals. These drugs clearly produce self-administration.

Dr. Mark Gold
Alcoholism & Addiction
October 1985

Hotly contested is the issue of whether the DEA prematurely scheduled a drug that was presumed to have great therapeutic value, a drug whose potential could not be realized unless research could continue unhampered.

Doonesbury

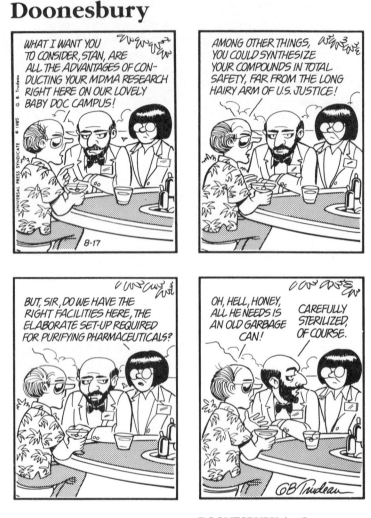

Greer and Grinspoon and that other fellow from Massachu-
setts—they mean well. They are compassionate, professional.
Maybe a little naive. They don't want to have to go through
FDA and get permission.

Dr. Frank Sapienza
DEA chemist
Washington, D.C.
November 1985

Drugs stay in your body. I only did MDMA once. Six hours
with my girlfriend, then we went out to dinner. I don't do a lot
of drugs because I don't know enough—they could be
f—ing you up in ways nobody knows. They shouldn't stop
research on drugs like MDMA. It's only by research that
people really know. Otherwise you think when they tell you
not to do it that they're on some punishment trip and only
goonies will be affected. Had I known about all the bad effects
of coke and some of the other drugs, I'd never have taken
them. I've seen successful people, intelligent people lose their
businesses, their homes, their families, wife and kids because
of cocaine. Just making a drug taboo won't stop people from
using it—hell, it just makes it more exciting. Like alcohol,
people have to know the facts and just how dangerous drugs
can be.

Member of Devo (rock band)
Los Angeles
November 1985

Many of the claims made about Ecstasy's psychotherapeutic
benefits were similarly made about LSD-25. At a 1965 conference on
LSD, Dr. Sidney Cohen summed up those claims:

—The patient's defensiveness is reduced and repressed memo-
ries and conflicting material are allowed to come forth. The
recall of these events is improved and the abreaction is
intense.

—The patient feels closer to the therapist and it is easier for
him to express his irrational feelings.

—Alertness is not impaired and insights are retained after the drug has worn off.

—There is a marked heightening of the patient's suggestibility . . . the judgmental attitude of the patient toward the experience itself is diminished. This can be helpful, for insights are accepted without reservations and seem much more valid than under nondrug conditions.

The fact that MDMA is now on Schedule I along with marijuana and all the other hallucinogens doesn't prevent research . . . There's hundreds of researchers and therapists licensed to work with marijuana in this country. That's what happened in 1966 when lots of people were sending away to Sandoz for free LSD . . . it was readily dispensed in a lot of therapeutic communities. When it became . . . a street problem, the government . . . said we're going to set up machinery to control all of this . . . so we can control these supplies and protect the rights of the subjects and insure that science will be done properly . . . Most of the people weren't interested in doing this kind of research. Instead, they went around the country saying that the government's down on LSD research—they're not supporting it. They won't let us do it. What they wanted to do was just continue to dispense it to their patients because their patients said they are better. If that was the criteria, then we would give all of our psychotherapeutic patients cocaine and heroin because they certainly would feel better and if we took it with them, we would certainly agree that it was improving things. This is not the way science proceeds and medical research proceeds. We need some kind of better description of what's going on here. The machinery exists for doing that—it's tedious as hell. I shuffled papers for a year and a half to get through that. But if you really want to do it, it can be done.

Dr. Ronald Siegel
Designer Drug Conference, UCLA
October 1985

There has been much speculation about the neurotoxicity of MDMA because of its chemical similarity to MDA and methamphetamine. MDA has been shown to destroy the serotonin-producing neurons in the brain. These cells play a direct role in regulating aggression, mood, sexual activity, sleep, and sensitivity to pain. MDA's effect on the serotonin system helps explain its purported power to enhance sexuality and give the user a feeling of peacefulness and conviviality. This is why it became known as the "love drug." Consequences of the lesions inflicted by the drug on the serotonin terminals in the brain are unknown.

> In the research we have available, the human treatment of "Adam" and "Ecstasy," you have a lot of data on toxicity, the adverse effects, the problems that we're seeing in patients; and this data is well presented by everybody who's promoting this drug as a new and wonderful drug and something that was available in treatment. But it's sort of glossed over when they make their legal presentations or media presentations . . . I'm still—and I really apologize to professionals involved with this because many of these professionals are my mentors, my predecessors, my professors at UC Medical Center who are involved in the testimony for these things—and looking at them and accepting and understanding what they're talking about—the pharmacology, the optical isomers and all that—I can understand what they're saying. But on a clinical standpoint for me who sits there and has to deal with sometimes what we call the casualties of substance abuse . . . I don't see that much difference between MDA . . . and MDMA which is one methyl group different . . . both drugs have the same type of effects when you equate their doses . . . similar toxicity, similar liabilities.
>
> Dr. Darryl Inaba
> Designer Drug Conference, UCLA
> October 1985

Methamphetamine has been shown to damage the cells producing dopamine in rat brains.

On October 4, 1985, Dr. Lewis Seiden of the University of Chicago submitted to the DEA preliminary results of the first controlled studies using MDMA in rats. He concluded after treating rats with multiple or single injections of MDMA that MDMA shows a greater depletion of serotonin after repeated doses. A single injection of MDMA may not be as toxic as MDA, but chronic treatment with MDMA appears to be more toxic than MDA. This study is controversial because it extrapolates from rats to humans.

Other evidence suggests that substantial depletion of serotonin may result in chronic depression—depression manifested not only by subjective feelings but also by adverse changes in sleep, appetite, sexual activity, and activity in general.

A central media figure in the Ecstasy controversy is thirty-two-year-old Rick Doblin, a building contractor from Sarasota, Florida. Like Timothy Leary, he is dedicated to establishing the safe use of psychedelics for "seekers of self-knowledge." He has taken MDMA at least twenty times and freely distributed it. He is raising money for a new pharmaceutical company that might conduct research on MDMA with hope of convincing the federal government that Ecstasy is not brain damaging. Should he receive a clean bill of health, his company would mass–produce MDMA for public distribution under the watchful eyes of doctors and therapists. "Return on investment could be very significant in the long run," says Mr. Doblin.

Given that Ecstasy isn't much of an aphrodisiac and doesn't pack the wallop of any number of other party drugs, it seems possible that it will be little more than a passing fad among "recreational" users—an ultimately disappointing street drug, something tried once because of all the hype and then discarded.

Joe Klein
New York Magazine
May 20, 1985

Dr. Ronald Siegel, speaking at the Designer Drug Conference at UCLA in October 1985, summed up the Ecstasy controversy in this way:

Unless you want to defoliate the entire planet and pave it over and outlaw the science of chemistry and cooking, you'll probably never stop the use of synthetic drugs or natural drugs in the search for ecstasy and altered states.

I've been in discussions with very prestigious jurists in America, Supreme Court Justices and law enforcement authorities at the highest levels who have recognized that we have a problem in that we are saying yes to alcohol and tobacco, which are the worst, and to coffee and caffeine and no to things like Ecstasy . . .

In another hundred years, perhaps, we'll have that world that Robert Silverberg envisioned. We'll be able to have a safe aspirin, a good five-cent intoxicant out there. Something better than alcohol and tobacco and marijuana and cocaine and Ecstasy. We don't have it now, but that's what the alchemists are looking for. And there is pharmaceutical research going on, even though they will deny it, for that kind of drug.

5 MPTP

◆ *Those of us who've gone to prison and tried all our lives to put out good dope, clean dope . . . are opposed to these new people [designer chemists] . . . Not too many cooks are combined in any type of organization . . . The purpose of the Council of Cooks is to get the toxic drugs off the street. To quit killing people. Cuz there's so much heat [law enforcement] behind manufacturing drugs. That heat came from people dying. If people were still laughing and joking and lollygagging and having a good time and nobody getting hurt . . . there wouldn't be so much heat . . .*

[Illicit] drugs are no different from the drugs the government puts out other than these pukes [designer chemists] putting out something that's not real. Misrepresenting themselves. Making a million dollars to boot. They don't have a right to that life. There's people that have been to prison three and four times coming up the ladder, working your way through here and there and it don't come easy. Some of us never make it. Some of us do . . .

"Let's Keep Drugs Clean" can definitely impact the black market. There's a lot of effort, a lot of arguments, a lot of boxing matches, a lot of friendships lost and friendships broken behind that particular idea because most of the people that are in the drug market have been to jail. They fall back into the convict code of "that's tellin.' " But at some point, you have to let that go and reach for a higher thing and that is ultimately that the drugs are gonna have to be kept clean or we're all just gonna have to get out of the business . . . We have our own police department. Our own way of handling things.

Convicted chemist/dealer/drug runner
January 1986

The Tragedies

Over the Fourth of July weekend, 1982, two brothers in Watson-ville, California, suffered paralysis after injecting a substance they thought was heroin. They had lain frozen for days in their apartment and would have starved to death if their mother hadn't stopped by to check on them.

Fifty miles to the north, a forty-two-year-old man and his twenty-six-year-old girlfriend mainlined a powder sold to them as "new heroin." The man hallucinated, something he had never done before while on narcotics. They had purchased four bindles of the drug from a Mountain View, California, drug dealer. The drug burned when they injected it into a vein—unlike real heroin. They shot up three bindles. On the Fourth of July, the girl woke up and couldn't get out of bed. The man felt stiff. The man grew worse while in jail four days later. He steadily froze up into a living statue.

He was admitted to the Santa Clara Valley Medical Center, where a doctor noticed movement in the man's fingertips. The doctor placed a pencil between the patient's fingers. The man wrote, "I don't know why or what is happening to me. I only know I can't move. I know what I want to do, but it just won't come out right."

Within weeks, Dr. William Langston, a Santa Clara neurologist, had seven paralyzed drug users under his care. Twenty other less advanced cases came to seek his help after news reports linked contaminated synthetic heroin selling on the street as the cause of what appeared to be advanced Parkinson's disease.

What had been sold to users was MPPP, a little-known derivative of the painkiller meperidine (Demerol). The MPPP was contami-nated with a toxic byproduct called MPTP, which is created during the faulty synthesis of MPPP. MPTP zeroes in on a section of the brain that controls movement and destroys the brain cells there. The initial batches of the so-called Demerol lookalike cooked up by the sloppy designer chemists contained almost pure MPTP.

By January 1985, the Centers for Disease Control (CDC), the Santa Clara Valley Medical Center in California, and the State of California Division of Health Services and Department of Alcohol and Drug Programs had collaborated in an effort to locate users of contaminated meperidine derivatives to inform them of the health risks linked to Parkinson's disease and to establish a long-range clinical follow-up on persons exposed to the neurotoxin. Approximately 400 young people were identified by the CDC as having used meperidine derivatives and their contaminants, which included MPPP, MPTP, PEPAOP, and PEPTP.

The complete findings of the CDC investigation, some of which follow, will be published in a book entitled *MPTP—A Neurotoxin Producing a Parkinsonian Syndrome,* edited by Markev, Castagnoli, Trevor, and Kopin, and published by Academic Press.

Viewed from outside California, the Parkinson's disease epidemic is considered a regional problem. A handful of researchers and the CDC, however, think otherwise. What horrifies researchers who are familiar with the investigation is the possibility that the contaminated meperidine derivatives were sold as speed or PCP or cocaine to unsuspecting users and the further possibility that they are still being sold as such. If so, thousands of users may be at risk.

In 1984 and 1985, the Drug Enforcement Administration busted two methamphetamine (speed) labs in which bootleg recipes of MPPP synthesis were recovered along with the necessary precursor chemicals needed to cook up the drugs. And in 1984, in Texas, a large-scale PCP lab was shut down at which meperidine derivatives were being synthesized.

Users who have been exposed to the toxic contaminants MPTP or PEPTP may not show neurodegenerative symptoms for several months or years. Potential victims may not recognize the symptoms of early-stage Parkinson's disease, which begin with barely detectable disturbances in motor movement, such as a tremor in the hands, loss of facial expression, or muscle stiffness.

At the time of this writing, two investigations are underway in New York City and Detroit involving narcotics users exhibiting Parkinsonism. In January 1986, the DEA confiscated red capsules testing positive for MPTP in Fort Lauderdale, Florida, which were being sold on the street as "painkillers."

Testimony: Dr. J. William Langston. Chairman Neurology Department, Santa Clara Valley Medical Center. San Jose, California.

What we think happened is a chemist in the Bay Area researched the Stanford Library until he found the very same report [and razored it out] that I think Barry Kidston [23-year-old graduate student suffering from Parkinsonism] used to make a Demerol lookalike which is called MPPP, which was uncontrolled and could be sold on the streets without any fear of prosecution . . . We began seeing young addicts that had literally frozen overnight. They looked like 70 or 80 years old with Parkinson's disease . . .

. . . a young woman was, I believe, 26 at the time she used this. It was the summer of 1982 and this was the first time she had experimented with I.V. (intravenous) drugs. She had used drugs before but never I.V. Over six days she lost interest, froze up and was taken to an emergency room as having hysterical paralysis. She was in that psychiatric unit for three weeks and then sent home and told it was all in her head. It was only when we identified the street heroin that a public health nurse watching the TV news recognized the symptoms (after a warning had been broadcast) and called us . . . This young woman had been frozen, unable to move at all, for six weeks when we saw her . . . If you put your ear on her chest, you could hear a faint sound. She was totally normal mentally . . .

We now are aware of over 400 young people who used these drugs in Northern California . . . We have gotten help from the Centers for Disease Control . . . When they left in January, I think they left almost in a state of retreat. They were finding so many new cases that we are overwhelmed. I think that we are touching the tip of the iceberg in Northern California.

Senate Subcommittee Hearings
July 18, 1985

The Poison

Meperidine, known by its trade name Demerol, is a synthetic narcotic used to control severe pain. It is controlled in Schedule II of the Controlled Substances Act. MPPP is a little-known derivative of meperidine that has been used in the manufacture of industrial chemicals. The DEA first identified MPPP on the illicit market in 1982. MPPP requires sophisticated lab procedures in its synthesis. If not produced under carefully controlled conditions, a neurotoxic by-product, MPTP, is produced.

In synthesizing MPPP there tends to be a lot of purifying and crystallization to get a product free of impurities. If shortcuts are taken in the heating process, something like a ten-hour reaction required at 30 degrees is instead hurried up to five hours at 40 degrees, then, as is true with MPPP, side reactions are sped up. In this particular case, MPTP is created by the high temperature shortcut. MPTP becomes the primary product. When NIDA synthesizes these compounds for researchers to test and work with, there is a great deal of crystallization for purity. The cruder street chemist is merely looking to produce a substance that will be MPPP active and if that means only 10% to 50% purity then that's all he's interested in . . . Without purifying and also risking shortcuts, there are countless possibilities for toxic compounds not yet tested.

Dr. Richard Hawks
Researcher, NIDA
October 1985

MPTP (1 methyl 4 phenyl 1,2,5,6 tetrahydropyridine) is neurotoxic to a group of cells in the brain known as the substantia nigra—the identical area damaged by Parkinson's disease. A few chemists working with MPTP during industrial operations have suffered Parkinsonian movement disorders resulting from either inhalation or absorption of the contaminant through the skin. The drug evaporates at room temperature in liquid form.

Abuse of MPPP was first reported in 1976, when a twenty-three year-old graduate student in Washington, D.C., was referred to the National Institute of Mental Health after exhibiting Parkinson's disease symptoms. A self-admitted addict, he had been injecting MPPP that he had manufactured for his personal use. It was later discovered that he had inadvertently produced MPTP through faulty lab procedures. MPTP was later linked to Parkinson's disease.

Since 1976, numerous samples of illicitly produced MPPP that contain the neurotoxic byproduct MPTP have been identified. Recently in Texas and California a second designer version of meperidine called PEPAOP has been identified. PEPAOP was contaminated with a byproduct called PEPTP, which has been linked to another neurodegenerative disease known as Huntington's Chorea, which causes spasmodic movements of the limbs and facial muscles.

The chemist didn't f— those people up. They did it to themselves. I mean if you're going to do drugs, use your f—ing head . . . No, I don't think they can get the guy [chemist] for directly doing it, but there's a lot of other things he's done wrong they can nail him on.

Former speedfreak
New York City
November 1985

Not many of them want to go in for examination and treatment, because they're addicts, and so they get along as best they can on the streets, or with their families.

Dr. James Ruttenber
High Times
October 1985

Me and my girlfriend split what we bought. She took hers home and I did mine by myself. When I tried it, it burned in my arm and other really weird things. I got really scared. I didn't do no more. I didn't tell anybody because I was afraid I'd get in trouble.

Female
First-stage Parkinson's disease
September 1986

A few people might see this tragedy as an argument to legalize the distribution of opiates so that incidents such as the MPTP syndrome can be avoided. It may be claimed that drug-dependent individuals have the right to quality, purified material to support their addiction. Realistically, it is impossible to protect a person who will not take the responsibility for protecting himself. In England, where heroin addicts are given sterile opiates and syringes, the incidence of hepatitis and bloodstream infections matches ours . . . Addicts tend to be careless or uncaring about these matters . . . Those who inject, smoke or swallow dubious substances have no self-esteem, no concept of future consequences, are extremely immature or self-destructive.

Dr. Sidney Cohen
Drug Abuse & Alcoholism Newsletter
September 1984

What's on the Street

MPPP, with its contaminant MPTP, is most often sold as heroin. Street names have included "synthetic heroin," "new heroin," and "synthetic Demerol." In Florida it was sold as an all-purpose "analgesic painkiller."

> If you try to make the Demerol analog [derivative], you will get some MPTP. You can absorb it. But what scares me the most is basically the formula is being sold on the streets to lay people and even a good chemist will get some MPTP. If we get amateur chemists using a xerox formula, God knows what will happen. Ironically, at the bottom of the xerox it says, "Warning, if made improperly or carelessly, this can damage your clients—see attached"; and they had a paper on Parkinson's attached. So they know.
>
> Dr. William Langston
> Senate Hearings
> July 1985

Physical Properties and Packaging

The meperidine derivatives are usually sold as white powders. An amber-colored powder with large granular-type crystals which was dissolved in water and taken intravenously has also been reported. Some users only snorted the drug. Red capsules selling as painkillers and testing positive for MPTP were reported in Florida in January 1986.

> MPPP has been mixed with cocaine and PCP. Users may not suspect or associate the acute symptoms of the Parkinson's disease with the drug. The cocaine was mixed for shooting and snorting. One of the people selling MPPP was also selling PCP.
>
> Dr. James Ruttenber
> Atlanta, Georgia
> January 1986

Distribution

Meperidine derivatives have been reported in California, Texas, Maryland, British Columbia, Michigan, Florida, and New York. According to the CDC report in April 1985, evidence suggests that meperidine derivatives are currently available in California and have been since the 1970s. A number of persons interviewed reported using meperidine derivatives in recent months; nine of them exhibited chronic symptoms of exposure to MPTP.

An epidemic of neurologic disease in narcotics users in the Netherlands in late 1981 and early 1982 is suspected to be meperidine derivative-related Parkinsonism.

As bootleg recipes for toxic designer heroins proliferate on the black market and the supply of contaminated synthetic narcotics threatens to increase, the question of a national drug monitoring system to test street drugs is raised.

My suggestion would be to take some of the best minds from around the scientific community, lawmakers and the pharmaceutical industry, get them together to look at all of the aspects to try to come up with a detailed program all the way from street monitoring to legal control.

Dr. William Langston
Senate Hearings
July 1985

I see no need for testing. If something's illegal, don't do it . . . If you test drugs, then you might as well make them legal. To me they are conflicting issues. I don't think we have unlimited wealth [to test drugs] and it's also immoral. I don't know where DEA stands—I don't want to speak for them. There are places to be compassionate and this is not it . . . I hope we don't get any street samples of MPTP. We don't even have a standard of it here. I just won't order it . . . Who needs it if it can cause Parkinson's disease? We don't want to be exposed to it . . . If we do [get samples], we'll have to do our jobs, I guess, and analyze it.

DEA chemist
Southern California
January 1986

We ought to set up a nationwide monitoring system to check for MPPP and MPTP. Drug users could mail in suspect drugs anonymously for testing. Drugs that test out negative for other active drugs from police evidence bins could be tested. Urine samples from methadone clinics could be tested.

> Dr. James Ruttenber
> Centers for Disease Control
> Atlanta, Georgia
> January 1986

If we must monitor drugs to prevent future death and disease, then why not make the drugs legal or allow controlled distribution and be assured that they are pharmaceutically pure? Ernest van den Haag argued in favor of the legalization of marijuana, cocaine, and heroin in a *Wall Street Journal* editorial August 8, 1985, to which one doctor responded:

I could go along with Prof. van den Haag's proposal, provided two amendments were added to the law: First, impairment of function due to inhalation, ingestion or injection of any substance shall not be a defense against criminal or civil liability. Second, no one who has become ill, impoverished or disabled due to use of such drugs shall be eligible for any assistance from funds obtained through taxes.

> John R. Ledbetter, Jr., M.D.
> Rogersville, Alabama

Black-Market Chemists and the Law

A good business investment. I made a lot of money.

> Clandestine chemist
> Linked to MPTP poisoning
> 1984

May God forgive him.

> Female
> End-stage Parkinson's disease
> 1984

Immediately after diagnosing the MPTP poisonings, Dr. William Langston of Santa Clara Valley Medical Hospital went to the news media during the summer of 1982 to warn drug users of the hazardous "new heroin" on the streets. The announcement encouraged an informant—who preferred to remain anonymous—to alert the Santa Clara County Sheriff's Department to a house in the county where suspicious chemicals were being delivered, possibly for the manufacture of illicit drugs. The informant supplied the packing list of chemicals, which included fifty gallons of ether, forty gallons of acetone, one hundred pounds of lithdride, and forty-four pounds of 1 methyl 4 piperidine. The precursors were all legal and were valued at about $10,000.

The county crime lab compared the list of chemicals with the preliminary analysis of a sample of "new heroin" given to Dr. Langston by two of his patients. The chemical list and the test results had enough in common for the sheriff to want to bust the lab. Getting a search warrant was another thing. No law, at that time, forbade the synthesis of meperidine-like drugs or the possession of the precursor chemicals. No judge would sign a search warrant. The sheriff, instead, got the fire department to conduct a fire inspection at the house so the sheriff could get a look inside.

The man who answered the door was clean-cut, intelligent, and cooperative. He explained that he was developing sno-cone flavorings and moisturizing creams. The lab was not operating at the time. A sample powder at the site was taken without the chemist's knowledge and given to a forensic lab for identification. Halle Weingarten was the forensic toxicologist at the Santa Clara County crime lab who fit the puzzle together after she remembered an obscure article written about a graduate student suffering from Parkinsonism after injecting his homemade meperidine lookalike. Analyses at the crime lab showed the sample to be the same substance used by the addicts suffering Parkinsonism. It was the identical "new heroin" with the MPTP contaminant. The fire officials gave the chemist a day to remove the hazardous chemicals. He did. End of story. He was beyond the reach of the law.

There was a media lid on the whole thing. Summer of '82 seven people around San Jose all turned up with Parkinson's disease. They found the dope. The dope was contaminated. Dr. Langston, the guy treating them, went on the air that week soon as he figured out what it was. Now you'd think that would have been picked up by the wire services. You'd think that would have gotten all around the world. Know why it didn't? Cuz the damn DEA didn't take and broadcast it to the skies. They put a media lid on it. The reason they did that is because as soon as the local cops found out about this poison dope on the street—they had a lab where the stuff was being cooked up and they knew about the lab in Morgan Hill, but not exactly what was going on, so the local cops at that point got into the lab, they say, by pretending to be fire inspectors and illegally copped some of the dope.

When the DEA heard about it from the Santa Clara County D.A. crime lab, they went and talked to the guy and got some dope too and the fact was you couldn't bust the guy because the local cops had f—ed it up and the DEA had f—ed it up and the whole bust was all f—ed up and so that's why they didn't make a big thing about warning people about this dope. There was no way the DEA was gonna look like they f—ed up this bust where this guy had poisoned seven people and put them all in the hospital for the rest of their lives. They [the chemists] kept on making it—it was incredible!

I got a couple of clippings from the local paper that people sent in. I went to look into what was happening and couldn't find out a damn thing. Local police couldn't tell me anything. That's another thing. For about a year or two after that, local police couldn't and wouldn't say anything about that whole incident because they said a federal investigation is pending. When I'd call the Feds, they wouldn't say anything either. So nobody was able to find out anything . . .

They've known about these people. They said we can't arrest them because the drugs weren't scheduled. Bullshit! They could arrest them but they couldn't arrest them for something big like manufacturing Schedule I's. They could arrest them under dippy little FDA mislabeling and procedural violations.* They could have arrested them. They could have identified them. They could have brought them to court. They might not have been able to put them away in jail, but they could have fined them and identified them to the community. They could have done that years ago and they never did. And that would have nullified these people. Those people would have had to change their names, go underground and I mean they would have had the Mob going after them!

Dean Latimer
New York City
November 1985

That calm, intelligent, cooperative gentleman in San Jose may have been the same individual arrested in October 1984 in Brownsville, Texas. According to DEA sources, authorities busted the clandestine lab of a fifty-year-old San Jose so-called attorney who pleaded guilty to charges of manufacturing, distributing, and possessing PCP. In addition to his large-scale PCP operation, his lab was synthesizing PEPAOP, another meperidine derivative, which was contaminated with a neurotoxin called PEPTP (which, as mentioned earlier, has been linked to Huntington's Chorea).

The attorney/manufacturer is presently serving a ten-year sentence for the manufacture and distribution of PCP. While in prison, he himself has exhibited symptoms of Parkinson's disease.

During 1984 and 1985, raids on two methamphetamine labs in California turned up copies of typewritten recipes for the synthesis of MPPP, literature references regarding the synthesis of meperidine derivatives, and the actual precursor chemicals for the synthesis.

---

* The chemist arrested for manufacturing the fentanyl analogs linked to several deaths has been indicted for violating FDA regulations.

I am convinced that there are different batches still being made
and being made by former associates of that guy in Brownsville. Other people in other cities. We have intelligence telling
us it's the same people—I can't reveal those sources . . . The
whole thing has frustrated people in law enforcement. It's
taken them offguard. The DEA was not prepared to deal with
it. They don't feel it's important and they are adamant about
believing it's not been seen since 1982. In general, law
enforcement's not interested. They can't target it. They have
no information. No knowledge. And informants on synthetics
are non-existent. Meanwhile, it's not clear who is responsible
for it. The Public Health Service? CDC can't get support.
Right now, one million dollars appropriated by Congress to
coordinate the federal effort for designer drugs has been held
up by the Office of Management and Budget.

Researcher
Centers for Disease Control
January 1986

Using emergency scheduling, the DEA placed MPPP and
PEPAOP into Schedule I effective August 12, 1985.

Dr. James Woodford, an Atlanta forensic toxicologist, and CDC
chemist Robert Vogt have developed a quick and inexpensive color
test for the neurotoxic MPTP byproduct. Chemists can check for
MPTP contamination in drug samples or urinalysis by using a
porcelain spot plate and the common Marquis reagent. It tests a
vivid red.

Effects on Users

The CDC conducted extensive interviews in 1985 with individuals
who had unknowingly used contaminated meperidine derivatives
misrepresented as heroin, cocaine, and PCP. The original seven
victims of MPTP poisoning suffering advanced Parkinson's disease
were excluded and not part of the following statistics. The median
age of individuals interviewed by the CDC was thirty-one years. Of
173 interviewed, eighty-three are considered in the report. Fifty-two
are male, thirty-one are female. Thirty-eight are Hispanic, thirty-six
are white, four are black, two Native Americans and other racial
groups. Common early-stage symptoms reported by those exposed

to less potent contaminated meperidine derivatives included numbness in the arms and legs, muscle stiffness and aches, jerking of limbs, and blurred vision.

The following acute effects were reported by users injecting the contaminated meperidine derivatives:

—severe burning in vein;

—metallic or medicinal taste in mouth;

—jerking of limbs;

—tightness, stiffness, aching, or freezing of muscles;

—problems with balance or coordination;

—numbness of extremities;

—loss of facial expression;

—increased oiliness of skin;

—difficulty opening eyes;

—blurred vision;

—shaking or tremors;

—difficulty speaking and swallowing;

—drooling;

—hallucinations; and

—excessive sweating.

The symptoms above considered unique to MPTP and other meperidine derivatives include the burning sensation on injection, blurred vision, a spacey, possibly hallucinogenic high, muscle jerks, and tremors.

The following were symptoms reported by users soon after injecting the drugs:

Symptoms	Number	Percentage
Burning on injection	64	77
Spacey "high"	62	75
Blurred vision	36	43
Metallic taste	33	40
Jerking of limbs	21	25
Slow movement	20	24
Shaking of extremities	19	23
Excessive sweating	18	22
Stiffness of muscles	17	20

The spacey, PCP-like high reported by users lasted a few hours or less. Parkinson's symptoms do not appear immediately because the MPTP is changed to another compound in the body, which then destroys nerve cells. That compound is the MPPP metabolite, MPP +, a breakdown product produced from MPTP by an enzyme called monoamine oxidase, or MAO.

The original victims of MPTP poisoning suffered extreme symptoms—some of them literally freezing up, because, it is believed, they had injected almost pure MPTP. Later street samples were diluted by the clandestine chemists manufacturing the meperidine derivatives (possibly after word got back of the drug's crippling effects).

Parkinson's symptoms don't usually appear until 80% of the cells in the substantia nigra, a section of the brain producing dopamine and responsible for motor movement, have been destroyed. A number of the users who were interviewed may have lost a smaller percentage of cells because of smaller doses. If these people started out with a 60% loss and lost another 20% in less than ten years through the normal process of aging, they could suffer from Parkinson's disease well before they might "normally" have done so. Neurological damage of brain cells by MPTP is irreversible and worsens with time.

Treatment and the Future

Parkinson's disease was first described by James Parkinson in 1817. Today, nearly half a million Americans suffer from the disease affecting one of every hundred over the age of sixty. Symptoms of the disease—rigidness, palsy, bent-over posture, difficulty in speaking—result from the death of nerve cells in a tiny area at the base of the brain called the substantia nigra—"black substance." The cells contain a dark pigment and are easily recognized in fresh-cut sections of a normal brain. These brain cells normally produce the neurotransmitter dopamine, which then stimulates an area higher up in the brain called the striatum, where the origins of voluntary movement have been traced. If the substantia nigra stops producing necessary amounts of dopamine (because of the dying nigra cells), movement slows down, muscles grow stiff and rigid, and eventually paralysis sets in. The nigra cells continue to die after the onset of Parkinson's disease.

L-dopa, a prescription drug, has been used as a temporary treatment. The brain chemically changes L-dopa into dopamine. As the disease progresses and fewer nigra cells are left to convert the L-dopa into dopamine, higher and higher doses of L-dopa are required, to a point where the L-dopa causes disabling and grossly disfiguring side effects—twisting, writhing movements known as dyskinesias.

We started these patients [victims of MPTP poisoning] out on L-dopa out of desperation . . . [a 26-year-old female] has her facial expression back. She can smile. The medication, L-dopa, probably saved her life. She would have died without it . . . However, the condition is permanent and anyone who knows Parkinson's knows that with time the efficiency of the treatment wears off and you get to a point where either the medicine wears off rapidly or you get intolerable side effects. At that point we say the therapeutic window is closed . . . You get too much movement instead of too little . . . [The patient] lost 50 pounds because of these movements, which are uncontrollable. A side effect of the medication. Usually we don't see it within five years. She got it within three weeks. You have to drop the medicine down. Then the patient freezes up and can't move.

Dr. William Langston
Senate Hearings
July 1985

After Dr. Langston and his associates established that MPTP was the active agent in the synthetic heroin poisonings that caused the Parkinson's symptoms, National Institute of Mental Health (NIMH) researchers started testing MPTP in monkeys. Within the body, the MPTP is broken down by an enzyme called monoamine oxidase, or MAO, which produces MPP+. MPTP cannot be converted into the brain-damaging MPP+ without the enzyme MAO.** Researchers found that if monkeys were given inhibitors to block the action of MAO, they would not develop Parkinsonism from MPTP.

**MAO may play its own deadly role in nerve cell damage. MAO catalyzes the oxidation of dopamine, a process that is believed to yield toxic byproducts such as peroxides and free radicals that destroy nerve cells.

Neurologists are now looking at MAO inhibitors as a treatment for Parkinsonism. Pargyline and Deprenyl are two such drugs. Dr. Langston has received approval from the U.S. Food and Drug Administration to test Deprenyl in Parkinson's disease victims. Researchers at NIMH and in Canada believe the MAO inhibitors can significantly retard the progression of the disease. When combined with L-dopa, the MAO inhibitors can help early-stage victims of the disease without debilitating side effects. Researchers are hopeful that in the future doctors will be able to detect neural damage that might lead to Parkinsonism at the preclinical stage, before the victim exhibits any symptoms. An early treatment could then be prescribed, preventing the disease. Dr. Langston and his colleagues at the University of British Columbia are using a special computerized X-ray technique called a PET scan which indicates diminished levels of dopamine in the brain by color changes.

MPTP and its metabolites strongly resemble certain herbicides and insecticides, such as paraquat. A high incidence of Parkinson's disease has been witnessed in rural areas where pesticides are frequently used. MPTP has also been thought to be an unwanted byproduct of manufacturing processes that is spontaneously created by common industrial chemicals. Both of these theories would account for the high incidence of Parkinson's disease in both rural and industrial areas.

Case History

At age fourteen, Barry Kidston was in a serious car accident in the Philippines and was treated with the painkiller Demerol. For the next several years he was in and out of trouble involving drugs.

In 1976, he was studying chemistry at George Washington University. He set up a basement laboratory at home, and after much research and experimentation, began synthesizing the Demerol derivative MPPP for his personal use.

After using his homemade painkiller MPPP for a brief period of time, he began to exhibit symptoms of Parkinson's disease. It was later discovered that he had mistakenly created the neurotoxic by-product MPTP. He died in 1978. The death certificate showed an overdose of cocaine and codeine. The following is excerpted from his mother's testimony during the Senate Subcommittee Hearings on Designer Drugs in July 1985:

> In January 1976, Barry was enrolled at GW with a major in chemistry . . . Our basement is not very large . . . He decided to make some—do some experiments. Basically, he told us they were for class, to help him in his classwork at GW, and also to try to develop a . . . nonaddicting Demerol . . . I guess he got into what we are now calling designer drugs . . . He had a little Aetna burner . . . He had one of those glass trays . . . I have a little note about that being washed in my dishwasher . . . He bought chemicals from mail order houses . . . He also went to various libraries and researched what he needed . . . He would xerox formulas and descriptions and pictures and bring them home and work on them. He worked really on top of my washing machine . . . He also used the dishwasher for washing various chemicals . . . We didn't realize what he was doing until . . . a boil erupted on his arm . . . He told the story that bees had stung him . . . He had dropped out of GW—he showed some signs of being lackadaisical around the house or not being enthusiastic about anything and then one day he couldn't bring his arms down out of the air. He was stiff. He was walking with a very peculiar gait . . . Barry was put in Sibley Hospital . . . He was completely catatonic. He was diagnosed a catatonic schizophrenic. They did give him electrical shock treatments . . . then there was a discussion . . . it could be a neurological problem. At that point we started getting into Parkinsonian syndrome . . . [I remember] he had made some batches . . . one of the batches he was anxious for—it wasn't quite ready . . . He injected himself with the medicine.

6 "Crystal"

◆ *We shut down this one meth lab—it was a mother and father
hooked on heroin and selling methamphetamine to support
their habit. The meth lab was set up between the baby's
room and the kitchen.*

Special agent
Bureau of Narcotics
October 1985

◆ *Crystal meth is 99% of our caseload. They've come up with
a new way of making it. They use ephedrine—a legal
precursor. We aren't even thinking about the other designer
drugs. We could bust a meth lab every day if we had the
manpower.*

Criminologist
San Diego, California
January 1986

◆ *She has a boyfriend and they love each other. She doesn't
want to take a chance infecting him. She's the junkie . . .
She was shooting coke and he was tooting crystal and coke.
She would toot and chew crystal on occasion . . . A lot of it
is ignorance and not willing to look at the damage it can do.
AIDS has become like a hammer on the top of the head of
any intelligent person who is at high risk—if you can reach
them. The junkie out on the street you can't reach.*

Psychotherapist
Beverly Hills, California
January 1986

Cheaper Highs

Methamphetamine. The gays call it "Crystal." The bikers call it "Crank." Everyone else knows it as "speed," and it's staging an unprecedented revival on the black market as the ultimate replacement drug for cocaine and heroin.

It is a drug so similar to cocaine in its euphoric effects that it fools all but the connoisseur. It is most commonly found where street cocaine is of poor quality, particularly in the Midwest. It is one of the few illicit drugs that can forestall withdrawal symptoms for the heroin addict. Because it is less expensive than cocaine or heroin on the street, readily available (except in some Eastern cities, where the heroin market is tightly controlled by organized crime), and of a purer quality (less adulterated, containing more active ingredient), and because it costs next to nothing to supply, it has become a multimillion-dollar industry, attracting hundreds of enterprising manufacturers, chemists, and dealers.

Besides being cheaper and less diluted than street cocaine, methamphetamine's most attractive property is its longer-lasting effects. Some Crack users are said to opt for the cheaper Crystal (methamphetamine) in desperation when their money runs out.

Curiously, a designer Crystal has appeared in recent months. It is a concentrated form of methamphetamine called "Glass" because it resembles tiny chunks of translucent glass. As Crack is to cocaine, Glass is to Crystal. Law enforcement chemists believe it is freebased Crystal for the user to smoke (few samples have become available to test). Others on the black market say it is merely a new way of making Crystal and is highly toxic because of contaminants.

Interview: Male psychotherapist. Late fifties. Working with PWAs (Persons With AIDS) and board member of AIDS Project.

I have used drugs in all manners, in all forms and all drugs. Heroin is the only drug I have not used . . . They know I've tooted, they know I've shot up, they know I've smoked, they know I've done it all. So they know I'm not just speaking as a clinician and that gives me credibility. They can't say to me "you don't know what it's like" because I *do* know . . . and they know it . . . and they can't bullshit me.

They come from different walks of life, different environmental and parental backgrounds . . . most of my clients, of course, are gay. Mostly men . . . I've worked with PWAs for five years since this first began . . . there are many who have not been in the fast lane and not used drugs . . . and have AIDS. Those who have AIDS who have not used drugs are a minority—but it's a large minority. I'm not talking 2%, I'm talking maybe 35%.

I see something like Crystal used for several reasons. One is certainly sexual because it enhances sexuality . . . Some feel that Crystal gives them a better kick than MDA. A better sexual high. A better socializing high. When I say socializing that means the party, the dancing, the discoing, the bopping around all night long . . . Most prefer Crystal. But it's going out. The gay community, and I'm generalizing, is really becoming aware of the dangers of drugs and taking a very strong stance about not using. I'm thinking about a group of five clients in the same crowd—they played together and they screwed together and they bopped together and every one of them has cleaned up. They haven't used in three or four months. Suddenly they are placing a value on themselves and their health and who they are . . . A lot of gay users are [quitting drugs] because they are so threatened, so impacted with the fear of AIDS.

Drugs and AIDS can equal each other in many ways. You lower your immune system. The more destruction you do to your system emotionally, physically, the more you're prone to disease. That didn't matter when it was just hepatitis. Didn't matter if it was the flu. But it matters when it's a life-threatening illness. This is the first time in history that they have been threatened. I mean they all know they can die from an overdose and they all know they can die from being killed by some pusher but they've never been threatened with such a hideous disease as AIDS . . .

It wasn't overnight that these people stopped using. A lot of things happened. There were several deaths in the group. They saw four, five, six people that were in their social life die. In one case, one man in the group has been ill and it might be the beginning of AIDS. It's not ARC [AIDS Related Condition] yet and we don't know what it is. But it's scary. And it's been very, very frightening.

Beverly Hills, California
January 1986

Interview: Biker. Early thirties. White. Large man. Heavily tattooed. Currently serving time for weapon's violation. Spent last twelve years in and out of state and federal penitentiaries.

I only use my own drugs. Methamphetamine . . . this right here's my life blood. I can operate good on methamphetamine. Sometimes I get a little bit wiggy when I get too much police on me . . . Lot of people like to shoot just for the needle. They really don't care what it is they're putting in their arm. If it's good meth, you'll use a brand new sterile syringe. You'll use hydrogen peroxide and water to clean around where you're gonna inject it and use A&D Ointment to put on you immediately after; and you'll throw the syringe away when you're done. You discount all chances of catching AIDS, catching any type of hepatitis. In my circle that's mandatory. I've already had hepatitis. I catch it again, I'm dead.

Best way to get rid of points is stick 'em in Coke cans and squish the can. That way it can't ever come out. I use once or twice a day. I tried my very best this time when I got out [of prison] to stay away from the needles. And I was. I was just eating rock Benzedrine—amphetamine sulfate which is a lot easier to make than meth. But before it could take effect on one occasion, I crashed my car . . . when I need instant wake-up, I need instant wake-up. So I go back to the other thing [shooting].

January 1986

Then and Now

The amphetamines are a large group of synthetic drugs which are remarkably similar to cocaine in their effects but longer-acting. Methamphetamine was synthesized in 1919, and was found to have properties similar to amphetamine as a central nervous system stimulant. It is sold today under the brand names Desoxyn and Methampex and is used to prevent narcolepsy, a rare disease which causes its victims to fall asleep repeatedly. It is also used to calm hyperactive children and to help improve their concentration.

Amphetamine was itself originally marketed in 1932 as Benzedrine, a nasal inhaler and decongestant. During World War II, the armed forces of America, Great Britain, Japan, and Germany were issued amphetamines to counteract fatigue, build confidence, improve alertness and performance, and maintain physical endurance.

During the next several years, use of amphetamines spread through the general population. During the 1960s, heroin addicts on the West Coast obtained prescriptions for methamphetamine, which they used in combination with heroin—the "speedball," or used to prevent withdrawal sickness when heroin was not available. As abuse became widespread, injectable methamphetamine (Methedrine ampules) were withdrawn from the commercial marketplace. Illicit "speed labs" surfaced primarily in Northern California as early as 1962 to meet a growing demand for the drug.

At that time, anti-LSD and anti-marijuana campaigns were said to have encouraged the conversion to speed. So much publicity was circulating about the toxic effects of LSD and marijuana that information about the truly disastrous effects of methamphetamine did not reach users who were experimenting with the drug for the first time. Speed was being sampled by marijuana smokers and LSD aficionados looking for a new drug kick and worried about the hazards of LSD and pot.

The damaging effects of speed provoked Allen Ginsberg to claim in the *LA Free Press* in 1965 that speed was "anti-social, paranoid-making, it's a drag, bad for your body, bad for your mind . . . a plague in the whole dope industry. All the nice gentle dope fiends are getting screwed up by the real horror, monster Frankenstein speedfreaks."

Publicity accompanying the soon-to-follow anti-speed campaigns merely helped to popularize the drug. This notion of popularizing drugs via anti-drug campaigns (including narcotics, marijuana, and LSD) is discussed at length in Edward M. Brecher's superb documentary study of the drug scene entitled *Licit and Illicit Drugs,* published in 1972 by Consumers Union Report.

Suddenly "speedfreaks" had replaced "acid-heads" and law enforcement immediately stepped up its activity to curtail the use of methamphetamine. Obtaining precursor chemicals for the illicit manufacture of speed became more and more difficult. Meanwhile, another stimulant, cocaine, was staging a comeback (having been replaced by amphetamines for nearly three decades). Cocaine smuggling flourished as cocaine became a fashionable, though expensive, stimulant to replace methamphetamine. By diluting the pure cocaine hydrochloride several times, black-market suppliers earned huge revenues, doubling, tripling, and quadrupling profits.

Early reports from the 1970s suggesting that cocaine was non-addictive and that "speed kills" facilitated the switch to this organic imported stimulant. During the late 1970s and 1980s, cocaine took the limelight as government manpower, money, and intelligence were directed in a concentrated effort to keep cocaine out of the country.

Like the swing of a pendulum, while law enforcement was cracking down on imported cocaine, the methamphetamine trade surged ahead in productivity as hundreds of labs popped up in Northern and Southern California, supplying a national distribution network.

We are the leading state in the nation in production of methamphetamines and the problem is growing worse all the time. These labs are everywhere. Our Sacramento field office can't seize them fast enough to keep up.

Robert Elsberg
Bureau of Narcotics
Lab Task Force
April 1986

Italians are making it on the East Coast and shipping it out here. I'd say it was the predominant drug being used on the street. Easily. Definitely a replacement for coke. For one, it's cheaper. It gets you higher longer for less.

Crank manufacturer
Los Angeles County Jail
January 1986

There hasn't been any Crank, any steady Crank around since the '60s in New York. No Crank. Out West—not here. I don't know what the fags do here. I imagine they do pharmaceutical stuff. I don't think the people who distribute the junk [heroin] allow meth on the market. Very conservative here. I mean you don't hear about big meth labs getting busted around here. Cocaine! Oh yeah, there's a hell of a lot of cocaine around here. What do we need with meth?

Former speedfreak
New York City
November 1985

Wherever heroin or cocaine are in short supply or too expensive for the user, methamphetamine becomes an acceptable alternate (with the exception of large, Mafia-controlled East Coast cities). Even where cocaine is plentiful, methamphetamine is sold as cocaine to inexperienced users who cannot tell the difference.

I know quite a few reformed heroin addicts that are now off into speed—which I see as a little bit better chance in life. At least they're not sitting with their chin on their chest and their eyes closing. At least they see the things that go by 'em. Maybe they won't understand 'em. Depends what kind of speed they're shooting . . . the dirtier the dope, the worse it affects the mind.

Convicted drug runner
Northern California
January 1986

More and more middle class users are doing meth instead of coke. They are doing it—snorting and shooting—because the quality is around 60%. The coke they're getting, by comparison, is a lot poorer quality and it's highly adulterated. Plus, they're paying more money for the coke. One half-gram is about $60. A quarter-gram of meth is about $25 but will go a lot further.

Detective
San Francisco Police Department
October 1985

As long as you're not killing somebody, they [the government] don't come down on you that hard. Now they got a serious war on drugs nationwide and it's because of these fools putting out drugs they don't care about. You say, "Hey man, you can't be puttin' out that stuff on the street cuz I met people that are on your drugs and they're dingy—they do a bit and they go off into some f—ing cold world." You know what they say? "Hey, it sells" or they say "we didn't have any left." I mean they sold all they could make! Cuz people don't know nothin' about dope. 95% of the people say they snorted cocaine have never *seen* cocaine.

Convicted drug runner
Northern California
January 1986

For the dealer misrepresenting methamphetamine as cocaine a substantial profit can be realized. Meth costs little to synthesize in inexpensive laboratory operations that can be set up and dismantled in a few days' time. In the methamphetamine trade there are fewer middlemen (dealers) diluting the product, so they realize a bigger profit. New techniques for synthesizing the drug using legal precursors have further encouraged black-market entrepreneurs in the methamphetamine trade.

> I was tired of no methamphetamine from 1970 to 1980. They [the law] got ten years their way. So we got five years of ours [1980-1985]. Now we'll see who the next five years goes to because they're never going to stop it again. But I do hope they continue to make laws outlawing phenyl-2-propanone, methylamine, phenylacetic acid and things like that. Because those are the known precursors of methamphetamine. I think they oughta take 'em all and outlaw every f—in' one of 'em. That would help [get rid of the bad chemists]. The rest of us just go back steps [synthesize their own precursors].
>
> Crank manufacturer
> California
> January 1986

What's on the Street

> The sores you see on Cranksters' faces are often caused by bad dope with a lot of byproduct.
>
> Narcotics detective
> Northern California
> October 1985

> We seized a bunch of methamphetamine that had been cut with strychnine and cyanide. Now I can't believe they are deliberately doing that. I think they just don't know what the hell they're doing.
>
> Narcotics detective
> Central California
> October 1985

Street names for methamphetamine include "Crystal," "Crank," "speed," "meth," "Glass," "D-Meth," and so on.

Physical Properties and Adulterants

Methamphetamine is most commonly sold as a white powder for shooting and snorting. "Glass" resembles translucent chunks of glass.

We've heard the reports about Glass but we haven't gotten any in the lab to test. I've been told it's freebased methamphetamine for smoking.

Forensic chemist
Los Angeles Sheriff's Department
June 1986

Meth [on the street] is pretty clean. Largely. Especially the last couple years. Percentage [of active ingredient] doesn't vary greatly. It is rarely less than 25%, and that is unusual and real dirt meth. 50% or more is good stuff. Sugar, lactose, cornstarch, ephedrine, pseudoephedrine are used as cut.

DEA chemist
San Diego, California
January 1986

Some of the methamphetamine seized recently in Southern California has been contaminated with belladonna, which results from faulty lab synthesis using atropine as a starting agent. Pharmaceutical belladonna has several different trade names and is used to reduce spasms of the digestive system, bladder, and urethra. Methamphetamine cut with belladonna can produce excessively rapid heartbeat and breathing, dizziness, fever, hallucinations, agitation, flushed face, and possible convulsions.

We have users coming in with swollen faces who have been doing Crystal or Crank. The byproducts are causing the swelling.

Dr. Darryl Inaba
Haight-Ashbury Free Medical Clinic
San Francisco
October 1985

I'm no street dealer. Get that straight right now. What they're doing out there is confusing everybody with all these mixtures—mixing hydrochloride, phosphate, and sulfate. People don't have any idea what they are getting . . . The rush is real good with this benzaldehyde—gets real strong with the females, for some reason a sort of sexual stimulant, heats 'em up in the crotch and they like that, though it's not methamphetamine like they think. That other stuff causing all the swelling in the face is cuz they cut the shit out of it with Epsom salts—makes you retain water. Benzaldehyde makes you break out in rashes all over your body. Pretty toxic chemical. That's just one of the problems.

When you look at methamphetamine, it's a white crystalline powder and nowhere in any book does it say it's clear or translucent. You'll see stuff coming out of Long Beach and Hollywood that's strictly translucent. They call it "Glass." That's dangerous stuff. It's not methamphetamine, it's benzaldehyde. Becoming real famous in Southern California.

> Crank manufacturer
> California
> January 1986

We confiscated a roomful of look-alike methamphetamine. Boxes and boxes of the stuff. Reason we're so opposed to it—a guy will take a hit, maybe mostly caffeine and he doesn't get much of a buzz the first time. So he takes another. Then another. Takes him five hits to really get off. And next time he goes out for a buy and this time he gets the real thing. What's he do? He takes five of 'em! We got another OD.

> Narcotics detective
> Inglewood, California
> December 1985

Labs, Chemists, and Dealers

Two months ago in Sacramento, a man was sentenced to prison for the clandestine manufacture and distribution of methamphetamine. Over a period of five years he had moved his secret laboratory operation from place to place in Northern

California. He seemed . . . to know when his operation was about to be seized. Narcotics agents pursued him from rented homes by the sea to mobile homes on secluded mountain property. Each time the agents moved in they found nothing more than . . . chemical waste where the lab had been hidden.

When he was finally arrested, agents found portions of his lab . . . in a makeshift treehouse on several acres of land. During investigation and lengthy interviews . . . it was learned . . . how the necessary chemicals were transported from chemical companies in California, Nevada, Oregon, and Washington in rented trucks to rented storage lockers. These lockers would be in close proximity to the secret laboratory locations. The lockers would then be utilized as 'stores' to be tapped as needed. This was all accomplished using precautionary measures such as radio scanners to monitor police frequencies, and in some instances surveillance cameras.

This man produced up to 15 to 20 pounds of high grade methamphetamine per week . . . He was proud of his business. His profits were immense. He drove Maserati and Porsche sports cars, lived in an expensive home in an affluent neighborhood . . . invested in stocks and paid cash for property . . . He said that when he was sent to prison this time (he had previously been incarcerated for kidnapping for ransom) . . . that he was optimistic about his reception inside prison . . . that he would be revered for his accomplishments as the chemist of a large-scale drug producing operation . . . that he was going to be a member of an elite group of brotherhood of criminals . . . Much to his surprise . . . prison is now full of enterprising clandestine drug chemists. The only distinction is that one is more knowledgeable than the other.

Dan Largent
Clandestine Task Force
California Senate Hearings
November 1985

The Western States Information Network (WSIN) received reports of more than 175 clandestine labs seized in California during 1985. Most experts believe that for every lab shut down, three more go undetected. At least 312 clandestine labs were taken down nationally. Most states do not participate in any information network gathering this type of statistic. For this reason the 312 figure appears to be a gross underestimation of labs raided. Texas and Arizona are believed to have thriving clandestine lab operations that ship PCP, methamphetamine, and MDMA (Ecstasy) throughout the country.

In 1983, the average methamphetamine lab produced an estimated eleven pounds a week. In 1984, the estimate increased to sixteen pounds. In 1985, the average methamphetamine lab produced twenty-four pounds of finished product each week. WSIN profiled the average methamphetamine manufacturer as a white male who is well-educated or has spent time learning chemistry from an experienced cooker. The chemistry lesson takes place most often in prison, where formulas are exchanged between inmates.

I know probably 50% of the chemists and manufacturers in the state [California] through the prison system and on the street. I pick every one of their brains to see where they're going, what they're doing, what they been doing. I have a direct line on certain things cuz people report things to me on the street. I do business all over the state.

Crank manufacturer
California
January 1986

Some of these people [users] are also very heavy dealers—that's how they support their habit . . . Two dealers (I know of) are planning to quit . . . no dealer retires happily. You either get busted, or you get robbed blind or you get murdered . . . The two people still dealing are making plans and putting money aside so carefully—I mean it used to be lines of coke would be out for everybody who came to visit . . . Right now it's a business they are into and stuck with until they can get enough money to get out.

Psychotherapist
Beverly Hills, California
January 1986

The chemist may have ties to outlaw motorcycle gangs who will supply him with the necessary precursor chemicals as well as protection and a marketplace for the finished product. Approximately twenty-four pounds of high-grade methamphetamine will sell on the black market for approximately half a million dollars.

The Heathens killed one of their boys for dealing PCP. Bikers will only deal meth. It's in their by-laws. God help your ass if you start up a meth lab without bikers knowing about it . . . they have a monopoly on the industry. Methamphetamine product is their way of life.

> Narcotics detective
> Inglewood, California
> November 1985

In 1975 we were making LSD, MDA, amphetamine sulfate . . . We used to make—a long time ago before my eyes were open to the damage—we probably manufactured more Angel Dust than anybody in the state. Got out of that business completely. We didn't allow anybody to be in that business. Saw bad things inside family circles. When you start seeing things like they can't answer the phone correctly with the simplest instruction—then you *know* something's wrong. I seen deaths.

> Convicted drug runner
> Northern California
> January 1986

Many of the labs now being seized are polydrug labs, with PCP cooking in one corner and methamphetamine in the other. The next development forecasted by law enforcement is for the manufacturers of PCP and speed to move into the business of manufacturing synthetic narcotics. Three speed and PCP labs taken down in recent months possessed formulas for the synthesis of synthetic heroin.

Effects on Users

Like other stimulants, methamphetamine produces euphoria, relieves fatigue, suppresses appetite, and reduces the need for sleep. The effects on the central nervous system and cardiovascular system are strikingly similar to cocaine. Users feel exhilarated with an overwhelming sense of well-being and intellectual acuity.

> They [AIDS patients] do Crystal because they want to forget.
> They are in pain. They are lonely. It temporarily makes them
> feel good. They haven't got much else.
>
> Counselor for AIDS patients
> Subsequently died from AIDS
> December 1985

When taken intravenously, the effect of Crystal is felt within seconds. Evidence suggests that impurities in the street methamphetamine produce the powerful rush or initial "kick," since pharmaceutical preparations do not produce as intense a reaction. As in cocaine use, there is the desire to recreate the initial rush and euphoria and the desire to avoid the inevitable comedown characterized by fatigue and depression. The methamphetamine high lasts four to six hours, considerably longer than cocaine.

Addiction liability is high, as the user quickly builds tolerance and increases his or her consumption, because of the drug's reinforcing aspects as well as the negative aftereffects.

> I did all this other dope. Then I found the one I really loved.
> Speed. Got strung out on speed. Only about four or five
> months. Week-and-a-half runs. Then sleep two or three days. I
> skin-popped it a few times just to see if it worked better than
> doing it orally. I usually snorted it or ate it. Mainly ate it.
> Pharmaceutical bullshit is what I usually had. Got tremen-
> dously strung out! Holy shit! Put myself through detox—I
> simply flew back home where I come from—400 miles away in
> the mountains where there was nothin'. Got myself stuck in a
> mountain cabin for three months. There was no dope for a
> few hundred miles. Matter of fact, had to walk eight miles to
> the nearest general store!
>
> Former speedfreak
> New York City
> November 1985

Adverse reactions depend on the user's sensitivity and tolerance to the drug. Common complaints include headaches, dizziness, confusion, agitation, nausea, and muscle aches and pains. As doses

increase and use escalates, bizarre behavior is manifested by paranoia, frequent mood changes, absorption in meaningless and repetitive tasks, and constant picking and scratching of the skin.
Methamphetamine psychosis is exhibited after prolonged chronic use
and is similar to cocaine psychosis, in which the user imagines he
sees and feels bugs and worms crawling on or under his skin.

> A friend of ours strung out on Crystal has twice jumped out
> his window. Last weekend it happened a third time and this
> time he broke his leg in the tree outside his window. Other
> than his Crystal habit he's making a decent living as a designer
> and, well, maybe this will settle him down.
>
> Actor
> Los Angeles
> October 1985

Long-term use results in physical deterioration, leaving the user
susceptible to infections, sores, and illness because of the lack of
food and sleep and the strain placed on the cardiovascular system.
In the 1980s the greatest risk taken by intravenous users of
methamphetamine is the potential contamination and the spread of
AIDS.

> Your speed, Crystal, methamphetamine . . . is found mostly in
> the homosexual and biker communities. There's a lot of this
> stuff exchanged for sexual favors. We've busted gay parties
> where there's been boxes of points and all the paraphernalia in
> case of overdose. Very conscientious. We are talking *prepared*.
> Then one party we bust really late—maybe 2 A.M. and
> everybody is tweaked. We knew one of the guys there had
> AIDS. We'd run into this guy before. Guess who-all is sharing
> the same syringe?
>
> Narcotics detective
> West Hollywood, California
> December 1985

> I got a call in the middle of the night from a former business
> associate. He begged me to come over to his house because he
> needed to talk to me—that it was urgent and he started crying

on the phone! So against my better judgment I got in my car and drove over there. When I got there all the lights were out. I was scared to death and I called out his name. I heard him. He was down in the basement! I went down the stairs and he was sitting in a corner . . . The place was a disaster—junk everywhere. He's lost a lot of weight and he's been sick. Anyway, he went on and on about god knows what and finally I had to get out of there. I mean, he'd been so successful in his business. I called a mutual friend the next day to tell him what happened and he said, "Didn't you know—he's shooting Crystal."

Businesswoman
Los Angeles
June 1986

After chronic use—injecting methamphetamine—I've known users who experienced symptoms of Huntington's Chorea. Sort of spastic movements like an arm shooting out or your head swiveling around or darting back over your shoulder. Very weird. They call them speed bumps. They go away after you quit the dope.

Former speedfreak
New York City
July 1986

In the spring of 1984, a number of admitted methamphetamine users who displayed bizarre body movements were treated at the University of California Medical Center in Sacramento, California. Several other similar cases were admitted to the Contra Costa County Hospital in Martinez, California, during the summer of 1984. Forty-eight patients exhibited either choreaform or chorea-athetoid movements. The characteristic choreaform movements included involuntary writhing of the trunk and involuntary movements of the upper extremities, neck, head, and tongue.

Cooking Up and the Law

One of the best ways for law enforcement to beat clandestine drug manufacturers is to control the chemicals needed to produce illicit drugs. The law therefore depends heavily on the cooperation of wholesale and retail chemical companies to inform on suspicious buys of certain chemicals used in the synthesis of drugs such as methamphetamine.

There are four common procedures for cooking up speed. The most popular involves a reaction of P-2-P (Phenyl-2-propanone), a Schedule II controlled substance, and methylamine in conjunction with ether, aluminum, methanol, and mercuric chloride. Using this procedure, a chemist can produce Crystal meth (methamphetamine hydrochloride) within five to eight hours. Tools of the trade— glassware and other apparatus—cost as little as $400. Cost of the chemicals is under $1,000.

Although this is the quickest procedure yielding the purest product, it is rife with hazards. P-2-P is toxic. Methylamine, when ignited, will allow water to burn (it is a 40% solution in water) and is extremely toxic. Ether can be explosive. Mercuric chloride is poisonous. Cleanup of the crude reaction before the procedure is complete involves the formation of noxious gases. The prospect of raiding one of these operations is spooky for detectives.

Right now we are suffering a 100% casualty rate with our officers taking down these labs . . . spotted lungs, liver disease, skin burns . . . The biggest danger is fire and explosion. A light switch can set off a roomful of chemicals. Most of these labs are found because they explode. Our second big problem is weapons: sawed-off shotguns, hand grenades, sticks of dynamite . . . and the booby-traps. The refrigerator wired to explode if opened. The light switch wired with a grenade. And then the short- and long-term effects of the chemicals them-selves. Last lab we took down, a meth lab, I got a headache like a nail driving through my skull. I stepped outside to sit down. I looked up and saw two of our men running back and forth inside the lab like a couple of fast-action Keystone cops, jabbering a mile a minute. They were stoned out of their minds!

There's the PCP you pick up on your clothes and shoes, the ether ready to explode, the lithium aluminum hydride will explode with a single drop of water—a million things. And it's gotten to the point we don't let our female officers go into the labs because of the effects the chemicals may have on women of child-bearing age.

Special agent
Clandestine Lab Seminar
California Narcotics Officers Association
San Francisco
October 1985

During February 1986, two DEA agents began undercover negotiations with a clandestine laboratory operator who alleged he was making 25 pounds of methamphetamine a week. The following is part of their case report:

During undercover negotiations at the chemist's laboratory site, which was located across the street from a grade school, there was a constant influx of users, "street people," entering the site and purchasing methamphetamine. Within approximately five minutes of injection, the abusers became pale, their eyes would water, and they would begin to shake . . . During one meeting, the chemist displayed a pint-sized bottle with a dark brown liquid. Inside of it he said was "meth oil" (methamphetamine base). When he took the lid off of the bottle, the agents noticed a strong smell, similar to that of an insecticide. The agents were ill for several weeks after this incident, displaying flu-like symptoms, i.e., headaches, cramps, nausea. The chemist would often bury his "meth oil" up to six to eight months at a time, and would add iodine as a preservative. He purchased "Thrust," an additive for gasoline, from which he said he could extract ether . . . Once the methamphetamine powder and the ether were mixed, brown specks appeared, which the chemist picked out, claiming they were impurities. The sophistication of the chemist's methods can be indicated by the items he used in his manufacture: a clothes' pressing iron, a hair dryer, Mr. Coffee filters and a turkey baster.

Special Report
Huntington's Chorea
Divisional Intelligence Unit
San Francisco Field Division
July 1986

Possessing and manufacturing methamphetamine can bring a fifteen-year sentence and a $250,000 fine. In January 1985, the California State Legislature prohibited the possession or sale of P-2-P, which is crucial to the above-discussed procedure for synthesizing methamphetamine. Meanwhile, clandestine chemists have developed new methods using legal precursors that can be easily purchased commercially.

The second most popular procedure and one which is gaining dramatically in popularity involves the reaction of hydroiodic acid, a particularly potent acid, red phosphorus and ephedrine in an extended controlled reaction . . . a cleanup series is done using fairly potent corrosives and solvents . . . In order to produce a pound of methamphetamine hydrochloride, the apparatus would cost about $400 while the chemical cost is approximately $1,000 . . . Nothing in the procedure is controlled or restricted . . . there are virtually no odors or toxic materials used.

Criminologist
Bureau of Forensic Services
California Senate Hearings
November 1985

With each new precursor restricted, the more ingenious chemists merely synthesize whatever was made illegal.

The local narcs busted [a street lab] in Contra Costra County and they found in this Crank laboratory—Crank and LSD laboratory—gobs and gobs of empty aluminum foil packages . . . street chemists learn they need aluminum trihydrate and so they just make their own.

Dr. Darryl Inaba
Designer Drug Conference, UCLA
October 1985

One of the biggest complaints from investigators is that they have a surplus of leads on clandestine operations, but not the manpower to go after them. Other law enforcement officials feel their hands are tied at the local level without wiretap authority and a bigger take on manufacturers' and dealers' assets.

We don't need any more regulations—we need manpower. We need more agents, more courts, and more prosecutors.

Narcotics detective
San Diego Police Department
November 1985

We have the people but we don't have the laws. We need a
state wiretap law and a streamlined asset seizure law.

> Group head
> Clandestine Labs
> Los Angeles Police Department
> November 1985

Under the Expanded Powers . . . we can seize financial assets,
vehicles, aircraft and boats obtained as proceeds from illegal
drug trafficking. Now it is time to add the authority to seize
other assets such as real property owned by illicit manufacturers and used to facilitate the production of controlled substances. It's high time we extended a little "pocketbook
justice."

> John Van de Kamp
> Attorney General, California
> California Senate Hearings
> November 1985

I'd love to drive around in that red Corvette [seized from drug
dealer] but I guess as narcs we'd just be too conspicuous.

> Narcotics detective
> Northern California
> October 1985

Current statistics show that nine out of every ten labs raided is a
Crystal meth lab. In the past five years, 1,811 labs have been taken
down by the DEA alone. Of those labs, 25% were in California. A
bill is currently being sponsored in the California Legislature
requiring mandatory prison sentences for drug manufacturers.

I just can't figure why they're [the law] comin' down so hard.
Let's just say Crystal catches on really big and we start puttin'
all the Colombian coke dealers out of business. What's wrong
with us local boys making a few bucks? And there's something
else. People can handle methamphetamine. You don't see meth
wrecking families and screwin' up athletes so they can't even
play. If they'd just get off my back.

> Crank manufacturer
> California
> May 1986

Stephen F. Higgins, director of the federal Bureau of Alcohol, Tobacco, and Firearms, said arrests in eighteen states were aimed at "outlaw" bikers involved in organized crime . . . Agents said arrests involving members of the Bandidos, Devil's Disciples, Nomads, Outlaws and Pagans gangs took place in Alabama, Arizona, Georgia, Idaho, Indiana, Massachusetts, Michigan, Minnesota, Nevada, New Hampshire, New Mexico, New York, Tennessee, and Texas. All told, officers seized ten sawed-off shotguns, ten submachine guns, twenty-six silencers, sixty-three rifles, one hundred pistols, 4,500 rounds of ammunition, four hand grenades, five pounds of dynamite, a stolen computer, fifteen stolen vehicles, and large quantities of cocaine, marijuana and PCP.

Los Angeles Times
March 28, 1986

A less-publicized hazard coming out of the hundreds of clandestine labs has been their toxic wastes. Chemicals used in the manufacture of Crystal meth are carcinogenic and some contain quantities of cyanide. Clandestine lab operations routinely dump their toxic by-products and wastes down toilets, where they end up in the sewage system (a system that doesn't test for these toxins). They are routinely dumped into our lakes and streams and along roadsides. As law enforcement is called upon again and again to investigate and then clean up these dumpsites, the taxpayer pays the ticket.

Interview: Convicted PCP chemist. Early thirties. White male. Small physique. Resembled a young college professor. Spoke at length about several of the designer drugs. The following are his edited comments on methamphetamine:

In 1968, at fifteen, I got my first start in the business. I'd already read most of the manuals and had moderate lab experience. I'd been fooling around with chemicals since I was a kid. I started out making mescaline homologues and selling them to my high school friends. Smalltime but everybody starts out smalltime. My lab setup cost maybe $2,000. I met a few dealers. The more contacts I made, the more dealers I met. By the early 1970s, I was turning out LSD, MDA, a little PCP, methamphetamine—you name it—it was a lively market.

One day I was approached by a big-time dealer affiliated with organized crime. He was looking for a quality chemist and a few investors to set up a big operation. We flew around the state talking to prospective investors—all organized crime. Everyone we met was eager to do business. For about $150,000 we set up a lab at a farm in rural Northern California.

I was clear upfront about the way I wanted to do business. I'd supply an exact amount of product every month for "x" number of dollars. That way everybody knows what's expected of them and you don't get these neurotic demands on your time. One thing I don't like is guys hanging around the lab with guns. It's very stressing. My associates, however, insisted on protecting the place. I was producing mostly methamphetamine at the time. Though I was earning several hundred thousand dollars, I finally had to get out from under the pressure. I can't work under tension. Not with guns on the place and people pressing me to up my quota.

State penitentiary
September 1985

7 "Dust"

 Used to be an old saying, "When ya got 'em by the balls, their hearts and minds follow." Well, that ain't the case with PCP.

Narcotics detective
Hollywood, California
February 1986

Who would, in their wildest imagination, predict that a dissociative anesthetic, which produced a high incidence of anesthetic emergence phenomena and was a drug which mimicked the primary symptoms of schizophrenia by distorting body image, would become the number one drug of abuse in the United States in 1978?

Edward F. Domino
"Neurobiology of Phencyclidine"
NIDA Research Monograph 21

Back in Favor

PCP (phencyclidine), most commonly known as Dust, first appeared on the streets in the 1960s after LSD-25 was controlled by the federal government. It quickly lost favor as a hallucinogen known for its "bad trips," which would linger for hours and cause users to become aggressive and violent. An unsuitable replacement for LSD, PCP all but disappeared from the streets.

Later in the 1970s, when PCP resurfaced not as a tablet but as a drug to smoke, it found favor with a new generation of drug users, who found the drug's dissociative effects appealing. Smoking a cigarette dipped in PCP also offered a cheap high that might last all day. PCP continues to be sold primarily to lower-income users in the city who ask for it by name and are familiar with its bizarre effects. Selling PCP and its derivatives outside that market is difficult because of the drug's bad reputation.

The name of the game for some PCP dealers with ready access to the drug is misrepresentation—selling it as something else—Ecstasy, cocaine, Crystal, MDA, psilocybin, LSD, and more commonly as THC (the active ingredient in marijuana). They target the inexperienced users or users eager to try a new trendy drug about which they know little—as was the case with Ecstasy.

A few "designer" PCP derivatives have been identified on the street in the past five years, including TCP, PCE, PCPY, PCC, and ketamine. In general, there appears to be less and less motivation on the black market to design new forms or derivatives of PCP, since PCP is itself a highly lucrative enterprise and few manufacturers involved in the trade fear the risk of getting caught. The general perception of those involved in the illicit drug trade is that it is a waste of the chemists' time and money to design new PCP derivatives merely to stay outside the reach of the law.

> **Interview:** Supermarket manager in small town in the Midwest. Early thirties. College educated. White male.
>
> I was out drinking beer at my favorite tavern in town. Met a guy—never saw him before. Sort of a college kid who talked up a real expertise on weed. I mean he knew everything about the best "sens"—how much it was selling for in different parts of the country, all the different crops coming into harvest . . . he was pretty funny . . . So then he shows me a vial with a bunch of tabs he says are THC. THC?! I couldn't believe it! He warned me it was 100% pure and if I take one I should watch out for diarrhea. I forget what I paid him, but I bought some and took one with my beer. Well, I remember sitting on the tavern throne for over twenty minutes shitting like a goose. And when I started out of the bathroom I swear I was wearing twenty-foot stilts and was afraid of smashing my head through the ceiling. Then as I'm trying to figure out how far away my legs are, I start hallucinating in all the primary colors. Well, it took me more than a half hour to walk up the street to get my friend at another bar who was supposed to give me a ride home. My arms and legs had gone numb and didn't exist and I was floating down the sidewalk—floating about fifty feet in the air. Later on, somebody told me it was PCP, not THC.
>
> *Wisconsin*
> *December 1985*

Interview: Convicted PCP chemist. Early thirties. White male.

I've been busted twice for manufacturing PCP, which is very odd since I prefer to stay away from the stuff. It's a devilish drug. There is a cyanide element in the compound which is toxic with overuse. Most users tend to overuse. Individuals go into convulsions. You get these people with superhuman powers want to kill twelve cops and can't be subdued. I only make it on special request. I'm in prison because I was set up on a sting operation.

Ninety-nine percent of the underground chemists are jackals who don't know what they're doing. All of my products, no matter what I'm making, are very pure. I have twenty years' experience and some of the most sophisticated university equipment at my disposal. I'm a metallurgist and pharmacologist.

Something you should know about the bona fide chemist's nature. We tend to be reclusive. We work in isolation in our laboratories for sometimes days on end. We sell to dealers, not to street people. Once the product is out of our hands, we can't be responsible for it. Dealers are always cutting the product with unimaginable adulterants. We can't be responsible for what happens to the user. I don't use. You can't use and also work in a chemical laboratory.

I keep my own records on people—mostly friends whom I've observed over the years taking certain drugs. I record hair loss, idiosyncrasies, neuroses . . . very interesting material.

Do I have sympathy for the users? Sure I do. More than ever after living with heroin addicts in the pen. They are sick individuals. I have a theory that certain individuals are predisposed to drugs from birth because of biochemical make-up in the brain. The brain causes the craving. They are sick. I turn out a clean, pure product. I don't feel guilty about that.

California state penitentiary
September 1985

PCP, phencyclidine, was originally developed in 1950 as an anesthetic for use with humans, but was abandoned after causing post-operative thought disturbances and agitation. Use was limited to veterinary purposes, and that stopped in 1979, when commercial production was halted as a consequence of more effective controls.

PCP was first identified on the street in the mid-1960s on the West Coast when it was called the Peace Pill. It quickly earned a bad reputation for causing delirium, aggression, and convulsions.

It became popular in the late 1970s as a powder to sprinkle on marijuana for smoking and attracted users intrigued by the drug's dissociative effects, which made users feel removed from their bodies and reality. In its pharmaceutically pure form, PCP is a white powder which dissolves in water. For the past five years it has been sold as tabs and powder, but most frequently as a liquid for dipping cigarettes.

Smoking PCP is preferred by users of the drug, who feel that they can better titrate the effects, which are immediate, and thus better control the dosage. It is a drug popular in low-income areas because it is cheap and the "high" is relatively long-lasting.

We've seen it heavy within our Latino population and also within our black population and some college dropout-type students that are heavy into PCP. It's another drug with designer analogs . . . You get a feeling where you are apart from your environment—that's the ideal ozone-tripping the PCP faddist likes. But it induces amnesia effects and has a high incidence of combative behavior. People get violent. I'm really afraid of it. One thing that gets me real excited in my practice is when I have to come to work and there's this big Samoan mother there, about 250 pounds. She comes up to me and says, "You gotta do something for my son." I say, "What's wrong with your son?" And I look over at a 350 pound guy sitting there and his eyes are nystagmus—they're jerking back and forth. And she says, "Oh, he been smoking that KJ, the Monsters, the Angel's Dust—he been smoking them Shermans." I look at the guy and he looks at me and he says, "I can do anything. I can jump off a building. I can break this door down!" Boy, I tell you, I'm afraid. It gets me real excited and I always slip near the door and say, "I'll send a counselor up here in just a second."

Dr. Darryl Inaba
Designer Drug Conference, UCLA
October 1985

What's on the Street

Street names for PCP currently used include "Wack," "Lovelies," "Superweed," "Kools," "Angel Dust," "Dust," "THC," and "Crystal," among others.

PCP is often misrepresented as something else. In 1985, PCP tested positive in street samples that sold as MDMA (Ecstasy), methamphetamine (speed or Crystal), LSD, THC, psilocybin, and cocaine.

We had a bunch of this Coke-T circulating. The dealers were telling their customers it was cocaine and THC. It was PCP. Dirty PCP. They were selling the by-waste from PCP. We saw some serious hospital cases.

Narcotics detective
Central California
October 1985

Ya hear that all the time—little dumb kids getting burnt. They give 'em pot and it's not really pot but celery sprayed with PCP . . . It's never more than speculation far as I'm concerned. I don't think kids are that stupid. Even kids know from word of mouth what drugs can do. And what PCP does to you is not what MDMA does to you. Kids are gonna know. So they do it once. Big deal. They don't come back. Dealers that do that with kids tend to get their legs broken . . . I've known lots of people who were so desperate they'd sell anything as anything. But when they're that desperate they don't go looking for little kids. Little kids don't buy from just anybody. Little kids generally tend to buy from people who are just a little bit older than them, people they know in the community.

Reporter
High Times
November 1985

Now that everybody is hip to these new designer drugs they go organic and think it's safe to buy stuff like psilocybin. This last batch we picked up was regular mushroom pieces from the store treated with PCP.

Narcotics detective
Northern California
October 1985

There are an estimated 125 derivatives of PCP. Five of those derivatives, including TCP, PCE, PCC, PHP, that have appeared on the street have been placed in Schedule I. Ketamine, a PCP derivative still used in medical practice, was recently linked to a string of rapes and robberies on the East Coast. The following item was published by the *New York Daily News.*

Scores of women have been subdued by a powerful animal anesthetic at metropolitan area nightspots during the last year, then raped by the men who drugged them . . . Ketamine . . . has been linked to rapes and robberies in New York, New Jersey, Connecticut . . . Victims voluntarily took a powdered form of the drug mistakenly believing it was cocaine . . . The investigation uncovered 14 confirmed cases in which rapists used ketamine to subdue their victims, and evidence of its use in "scores" of other attacks.

New York Daily News
November 1985

Subsequent investigations were unable to confirm all the cases. One man was convicted of raping two women. The substance involved in the case was alleged to have been ketamine.

This Designer Drug thing is really selling big in the media . . . Rapists dosing women's drinks [with ketamine] so they get all vegged out and then they rape them. Prostitutes are supposedly putting it in clients' drinks, in their Johns' drinks, so they can roll their Johns . . . Thing is, if they *are* doing it, it's dangerous as hell. Ketamine and alcohol have a real synergistic effect . . . why aren't people dying? Turning blue and dropping dead? My guess is it's not Ketamine. There aren't any lab tests but I think it's PCP . . . I've heard stories about joints laced with PCP and the girl gets all vegged . . . I'm sure that's what this is—Angel Dust.

Reporter
High Times
November 1985

Packaging and Price

In liquid form, PCP is most often sold by the ounce or half-ounce in vanilla and almond extract bottles. It sells for approximately $150 to $200 per ounce in California and $500 for the same amount in Washington, D.C., and New York. It is usually a peagreen or yellowish color and has the odor of dirty diapers.

Users buy liquid PCP to dip cigarettes or joints into or can buy predipped "Kool" cigarettes which sell for $20 each. Sherman Brown cigarettes, called "Sherms," are made in England and are also sold predipped. Unlike American cigarettes, they contain no saltpeter, which is used to keep cigarettes burning. The brown color of the Sherms helps disguise the stain of PCP. Sherman Browns cost $30 predipped and $15 for half a stick.

Lovelies are handmade cigarettes made from treated plant material, which is sold in bindles ranging in price from $5 to $30, depending on the plant material, which can be tobacco, marijuana, or parsley.

Baby bottles have been used to store PCP. Rinsing it out is not enough. There's been enough PCP left to kill a baby.

Emergency room physician
Los Angeles
October 1985

In rock crystal form, PCP resembles cocaine but has a yellow tint. A gram may sell for $80 to $135, a half-gram for $50.

In January 1986, CBS reported a new street drug called "Wack" sold in Dallas, where emergency room admissions linked to the drug averaged seven cases a day. The hospital admissions were all primary school children who had smoked the drug, which tested positive for PCP, formaldehyde, and a common roach spray.

As of July 1986, the newest trend to hit the East Coast has come to be known as Space Base—Crack plus PCP. It is most popular with inner city black youths. The combination of the two drugs produces powerful changes in mood and energy with a loss of contact with reality.

We have seen kids (on Space Base) who not only thought someone was following them but tried to kill the objects of their paranoia.

Dr. Mark Gold
Fair Oaks Hospital
Summit, New Jersey
July 1986

Effects on Users

In small doses, PCP produces a "drunken" state with numbness of the extremities. In moderate doses, PCP produces analgesia and anesthesia—insensitivity to pain and partial loss of feeling and sensation. It also produces a state of mind resembling sensory isolation. In moderate doses, PCP also produces a condition of suspended animation and loss of voluntary motion, in which the arms and legs remain in whatever position they are placed. In large doses, PCP produces convulsions.

The gangs use it all the time. It gives the feeling of omnipotence. It dulls pain. It might even remove it completely, considering what a subject will do to resist arrest. We have something like 80% of our gang-related homicides are PCP-related. Mostly Hispanics and blacks.

Narcotics detective
Los Angeles Police Department
October 1985

A South-Central Los Angeles man, fleeing a drug treatment center while allegedly under the influence of PCP, was arrested Tuesday after he ran down a teen-age girl, broke into his ex-wife's home and beat and choked his 2-year-old son . . . His son . . . was in critical condition at Martin Luther King Jr. Drew Medical Center . . . Also in critical condition . . . was the 16-year-old pedestrian . . .

[The man] had been driven to the . . . Health Center by his parents, apparently because he had been acting strangely while under the influence of the drug. [He] bolted, taking the car, . . . hit another auto . . . drove on, striking the pedestrian a

few blocks away, then hitting a light post . . . ran to the
nearby home of his ex-wife . . . broke through a front
window, grabbed the boy and jumped through a closed rear
window . . . attacked the baby, but his wife intervened,
wrestling the boy away and throwing the child into the back
seat of a car driven by an elderly woman who lived on the
block. [The man] jumped into the car, locked the doors and
began to choke the child . . . A passing Los Angeles police
traffic division officer spotted the incident and summoned half
a dozen other officers, who broke into the neighbor's car . . .
and rescued the boy.

Los Angeles Times
February 19, 1986

Users of PCP report both positive and negative subjective effects.
Many like the drug because they claim to experience a heightened
sensitivity to outside stimuli; they feel dissociated from the world
around them; they feel better because the drug acts as a stimulant.
They also feel mildly inebriated, as if they had been drinking alcohol.
The combination of stimulant and depressant is seen as a welcome
escape for the user, except when accompanied by uncontrolled
hallucinations, which is a common complaint. Other negative effects
include the feeling of paranoia, disorientation, aggression, and
confusion.

I've had ten bad trips in maybe three years. That's having too
many hallucinations. When I tell my dealer he always says the
new stuff will be better but it's never guaranteed . . . I always
buy from the same dealer until he gets busted, then find
somebody new. I've never been hospitalized for any of the bad
trips. Bad trips are unavoidable. Everyone reacts differently
. . . PCP enhances my artwork. I'm an artist. I usually smoke
with friends. My [gay] lover shoots heroin as her drug of
choice. I pay $100 for a half ounce [of liquid PCP]. Maybe
smoke three Kools a day.

White female
Los Angeles
December 1985

Note, in reference to the interview above: Three Kools (cigarettes dipped in PCP) far exceed a normal dosage. This was said in defense of the large amount of PCP confiscated from her to be used as evidence of intent to distribute. She seemed an unlikely PCP user coming from an affluent family, remarkably attractive, self-possessed and talented. She was interviewed in the presence of a detective.

Overdose and panic reactions are most often seen in first-time users who have taken PCP by mistake. In 1985, users who took large doses of PCP thinking it was cocaine or MDMA (Ecstasy) were hospitalized on the West Coast and in the Midwest.

We snorted it in lines like coke. I did one line. So did Ray. But Larry, he did about three lines. I don't know why because it hurt like a son-of-a-bitch. He was totally out of it and we put him in the back of the pick-up. What I remember though is Ray who went nuts and got really violent. He wanted to beat the shit out of everybody including myself. All you could do was stay away from him. He kept running around the truck looking for his twelve-gauge hitting anybody was in his way. Don't ask me how we all got home.

White male, mid-twenties
Minnesota
November 1985

The following is a list of physical and psychological symptoms encountered in emergency room settings.

At low doses:

—agitation and excitement

—gross incoordination

—blank stare appearance

—catatonic rigidity

—inability to speak

—horizontal or vertical nystagmus (rapid involuntary vibration of the eyeballs)

—loss of response to a pinprick

—flushing

—profuse perspiration

At moderate doses:

> —coma or stupor
>
> —eyes remain open
>
> —pupils in midposition
>
> —nystagmus
>
> —vomiting
>
> —hypersalivation
>
> —shivering
>
> —fever

At higher doses:

> —prolonged coma
>
> —eyes closed
>
> —hypertension
>
> —convulsions

Treatment

Most clinicians recommend placing the patient in an isolated environment. All outside stimulation should be kept to a minimum to reduce paranoia, anxiety, and violent behavior. Treatment of respiratory depression, convulsions, and coma need full life-support systems in an intensive-care unit.

> I wish I'd known five years ago what I know now. I could have prevented a lot of damage. Hell, you just throw a blanket over their head—cut off all outside stimuli and keep 'em quiet.
>> Narcotics detective
>> Hollywood, California
>> January 1986

Dr. Darryl Inaba of the Haight-Ashbury Free Medical Clinic talks about his clinic's treatment of PCP overdose victims.

They are violent. They are unpredictable in their behavior and they are superstrong. Because PCP blocks out any kind of sensory input into the brain, you have uninhibited muscular activity so they *are* stronger than normal, can jump higher than normal, they can beat up all these cops . . . When a person comes in under that violent mixture, we gang 'em! Everybody jumps on him. Grabs a leg. Grabs a head. I splint the arm . . . and we start chemically hitting them up cuz we can't control this person physically; we have to chemically restrain them.

We usually put them in a coma and it's dangerous. I wouldn't do it unless you're with a full medical team . . . We use either Haldol [haloperidol] or high doses of Valium. More often we use high doses of Valium first intravenously, slowly and carefully until we get that person functional or in a coma and then we have to breathe for them.

We also acidify the urine . . . We start dosing them with high doses of Vitamin C—bring in the cranberry juice. Sometimes we'll even use a chemical called ammonium chloride to change their urine to be more acid and get that PCP circulating out of their system . . . and we've gone as far as to administer three times a day ascorbital-activated charcoal—we make up a little soup of activated charcoal and ascorbital and make them drink it and as PCP recirculates out of the brain into the stomach—it likes to go to the stomach and then into the intestine where it's reabsorbed again—at least when it gets into the stomach and intestine, the activated charcoal is going to suck it up and they're going to pass it out this time . . . it is the most difficult drug abuse treatment.

Dr. Darryl Inaba
Designer Drug Conference, UCLA
October 1985

The molecule is rigid and stable and hard to eliminate from the body. It is almost identical to the Agent Orange dioxin.

Dr. Ronald Linder
California Narcotics Officers Association
San Francisco
October 1985

For chronic PCP users seeking treatment, complete abstinence from the drug for as long as a year is necessary before health professionals can assess the damage—measuring fluctuating levels of PCP in the body and the unpredictable effects on recovering users.

PCP has the capacity to recirculate. It has the capacity to be stored in fat . . . kids tell me that! They say what they do is— after they smoke some Killer or some Monsters and they're starting to come down from it, they jump on the floor and do a whole bunch of push-ups and get high again because they mobilize the fat . . . the PCP is going to be in their systems a hell of a long time . . . the metabolites of chemicals are still within the fats in your brain.

Dr. Darryl Inaba
Designer Drug Conference, UCLA
October 1985

PCP and Schizophrenia

Schizophrenia is a psychotic disorder characterized by loss of contact with the environment and a disintegration of personality expressed by chaotic feelings, thought, and behavior. PCP psychosis has been compared to schizophrenia for years because of the similarity in behavior patterns. For example, users display autistic and delusional thinking not unlike schizophrenics (see Luby in Bibliography).

In an experiment in which LSD and PCP were given to hospitalized schizophrenics, the LSD caused no more adverse effects than in normal subjects. But when PCP was administered, the patients showed "extreme exacerbation of their psychoses; the reaction persisted for up to six weeks" (see Luisada in Bibliography).

In late 1985, a dramatic discovery was made when researchers identified the brain receptors for PCP. Scientists from the University of Maryland who had been researching PCP since 1980 isolated the biochemical process by which PCP disrupts the nervous system and causes irrational and violent behavior. "We can correlate cellular activity at the molecular level with behavior in man. I can't begin to tell you all the doors it opens," said Dr. Mordecai P. Blaustein, physiology chairman and head of the research project.

The findings of Dr. Blaustein and his associates, Dieter K. Bartschat and Roger G. Sorensen, were published in the January 1986 issue of the *Proceedings of the National Academy of Sciences.* The findings included the discovery that PCP binds with certain protein molecules, blocking potassium channels in nerve-cell membranes. PCP then forces the release of large numbers of neurotransmitters, causing the disruption of normal transmission.

Because PCP psychosis so closely resembles schizophrenia, which afflicts more than two million Americans, the research could lead to new antipsychotic drugs for treating schizophrenia and PCP abusers without the adverse side effects of drugs currently used.

PCP and the Unborn

Incidence of drug abuse by pregnant women is escalating at an alarming pace. Because there is little literature on the subject, many pregnant women are unaware of the damage being done to their unborn children. Recent studies on babies exposed to PCP during pregnancy indicate central nervous system disorders.

> Typically they [the babies exposed to PCP] are very alert, very active babies. Their mothers often think they are smarter. They hold their heads up faster . . . But, in fact, it is abnormal behavior. Although we aren't sure why, the tone of the muscles in the head is of the kind that we see in [children with] cerebral palsy.
>
> Dr. Xylina Bean
> Neonatologist
> *Los Angeles Times*
> December 5, 1985

At six months of age, according to Dr. Judy Howard, medical director of UCLA's Suspected Child Abuse and Neglect Team, the babies exhibit jitteriness and agitation seen at birth. At nine months, the babies cannot understand how their hands work. By twelve months, the IQs of these babies begin to drop, according to a study conducted by Dr. Willis Wingert, director of Pediatric Ambulatory Services at USC Medical Center in Los Angeles. By 20 to 24 months, the babies cannot coordinate their tongues to form words.

If one considers the dissociative effects of PCP experienced by adults who sometimes claim not to know where their arms and legs are, the same could be happening to these babies who are unable to coordinate their limbs, unable to use their hands because they may not see them connected to their body, unable to walk because they appear not to know where their legs are.

PCP is a drug that stays in your system for a hell of a long time . . . [we have] a case of a boy born to a PCP dependent mother. Kid is five years old and still has 72 nanograms per ml blood level PCP in his system. It's just not leaving his body at all.

Dr. Darryl Inaba
Designer Drug Conference, UCLA
October 1985

PCP Chemists and the Law

PCP labs proliferate in the ghetto. It's the fastest way to a Cutless Supreme. It's a business. A means of making money in the ghetto. The drug is inexpensive to make, any amateur can do it, and it's relatively cheap to buy.

Forensic chemist
Los Angeles County
October 1985

PCP synthesis involves a two-step procedure, and the drug is easy and inexpensive to make. It involves, first, the formation of an intermediate compound called PCC and, second, the conversion of that to PCP using a chemical solution called a Grignard reagent. The synthesis of PCC is usually an overnight process, while making the reagent and converting PCC to PCP can be done in less than two hours.

The cost of the chemicals (excluding piperidine) and apparatus is less than $100 to cook up a gallon of PCP. Piperidine has a street value of $1,000 or more per gallon. Often, three locations will be used: one will make the PCC, another will make the Grignard reagent, and they will meet together at a third location to make the PCP.

Dangers of fire, explosion or toxicity are found throughout this procedure. Potassium or sodium cyanide is used in making the PCC which itself contains a substantial amount of cyanide. Ether, a highly flammable material, is used throughout. The Grignard reagent is a chemical liquid that is so reactive that it can explode when exposed to water.

Criminologist
California Senate Hearings
January 1986

A 30-gallon drum of cyanide and eight gallons of PCP with an estimated street value of $1.2 million were found in a South-Central Los Angeles house Thursday after fire inspectors went there to check out reports that the cluttered backyard was a fire hazard.

Los Angeles Times
February 28, 1986

There are two types of PCP manufacturers. The small-time operators cook up small batches for local distribution. They make the mistake of selling their product retail, opening themselves up to a number of potential informers. The second type of manufacturer deals in large, wholesale quantities that are usually shipped elsewhere in the country. They sell to one main distributor, who then sells to another distributor, followed by a network of dealers and subdealers. The chance of a big-time wholesaler being shut down is rare. There are no street informants who know who the big guys are. A good source of information for law enforcement are the chemical companies selling to the wholesalers. But these chemical wholesalers are unwilling to inform on their clients, from whom they are earning large tax-free profits, sometimes marking up merchandise 200% for sale to the black market.

We took down eight PCP labs in an investigation involving three chemical companies. The companies were under one head and they supplied precursor chemicals [for making PCP] to these labs. It was 90% of their business. We let the eight labs go because we had a bigger case against the chemical company.

The PCP labs individually were putting out between 5 and 50 gallons of PCP a day. Always in liquid form. Purity ranged from 125 mc/ml to 50 mc/ml. Rarely less. They produced only PCP. No analogs. Quality stuff. The labs were light-weights. The heavies are much smarter and know how we operate. They stockpile their chemicals, for instance. Sit on them for a while. The amateurs just buy up what they need and immediately go to work in the lab. The heavies deal with a few select trusted associates and they manufacture in huge quantities. They sell to a distributor who then sells to dealers who sell to other dealers at street level. The probability of a dealer or user informing on them is extremely rare. They don't know who they are.

Seventy percent of our caseload is PCP. Much of what is made in California is shipped to other parts of the country. It's in demand.

DEA Group supervisor
Los Angeles
October 1985

Los Angeles is the PCP capital of the world. The chemicals can legally and easily be purchased in California. More labs are cropping up in more remote areas where the odors can't be detected and there's minimal law enforcement coverage . . . We [local boys] work differently from the Feds. What it takes them a year to do, we can knock out in 90 days. I don't want to have to go to the Feds every time we have a big case . . . We put these chemical companies out of business and we saw a significant drop in PCP availability on the street [June 1985]. This is the first time in my sixteen years in law enforcement where I've seen a direct effect.

Group supervisor
Los Angeles Police Department
November 1985

PCP is currently controlled in Schedule I of the Controlled Substances Act alongside such drugs as heroin and MDA. Placing all potential derivatives of PCP in Schedule I will probably be as effective as outlawing PCP has been. Laws don't regulate the sale of PCP. Demand does.

In the case of phencyclidine [PCP], we have played cat and mouse with illicit manufacturers for a number of years, addressing each new analog of the drug as it surfaced on the street. From this we have learned that pursuing individual corrective legislation is simply too cumbersome and slow to adequately protect the public . . . as of this Monday we heard of a new analog of PCP. We are again playing cat and mouse.

Mr. Randy Rossi
California Department of Justice
Senate Hearings
July 1985

One of the biggest hazards for investigating officers is the risk of contamination when a clandestine lab is taken down. Detectives and agents are exposed to the toxic chemicals used to make PCP as well as to PCP itself, which can be inhaled or absorbed through the skin during the chaos of a drug bust. Symptoms reported by investigating officers after exposure to PCP during lab raids include drunkenness, hyperactiveness, headaches, skin rashes, elevated heart rate, confusion, short-term memory loss, aggressiveness, and hallucinations.

PCP is cumulative in nature, staying in the body for an unknown length of time. Female officers exposed to PCP have, at a later date, passed PCP to their unborn children, according to testimony by experts from the Bureau of Narcotics given at the California Senate Hearings.

The following is excerpted from a talk given by a special agent in charge of a clandestine lab task force. He was instructing a class of narcotic detectives attending the California Narcotics Officers' Convention.

At the smell of ether please, please do not throw a f—ing flashbang through the window as the roof will blow off and *you'll* have to put it back on! More and more local law enforcement are using Swat Teams with no narcotic background.

Never underestimate the "glass of water" in the subject's hand. We've had too many officers hit with hydrochloric acid, burned with methylamine, or had PCP thrown in their face—it won't kill you but I guarantee you'll never be the same.

Throwing a light switch, let alone discharging a gun in a strong ether atmosphere will blow the whole works up . . .

Wash thoroughly after leaving the site and don't even pick your nose . . . one officer picked up PCP on the soles of his shoes during a bust. He went home and unknowingly tracked it on the carpet where the baby was crawling around.

Don't drink after a lab bust. Breathing the air can later have a synergistic effect when drinking alcohol. Watch for your partner. You have a man down in a lab when a fire breaks out I can tell you right now no fireman will go in after him. Nobody goes into a lab where there's a fire.

If you can't get protective gloves and clothing and face shields, if your department or the higher-ups don't care enough about their people to protect them, then I say "screw 'em."

At a 1985 California Senate subcommittee hearing on clandestine labs, hours of testimony detailed the casualties suffered by investigating officers in the line of duty; the countless hours of nighttime and weekend surveillance required for a bust; and the subsequent obstacles arresting officers face in the court system—the seemingly endless frustration to get a conviction. Hearing this, a state political representative responded:

I find this entire business of designer drugs just shocking, just unbelievable. I mean every Californian should have been here to hear this . . . But now tell me, Detective ____ , have you or any of your men written letters to your legislators or organized any letter-writing campaigns to try and get these new laws you want—because, you know, that's how things get done.

Arnold Trebach, a drug policy expert at the American University in Washington, D.C., said in the June 20, 1986, issue of the *Wall Street Journal,* "Most of the leading policy makers and legislators are utter ignoramuses when it comes to the drug issue."

In the same article, Mark Kleiman, a research fellow in criminal justice at Harvard's Kennedy School of Government and a former Reagan administration Justice Department official, said, "Politicians love to talk about this issue, but they talk about it in a way that is totally remote from any attempt to make sensible drug policy."

Congress recently passed legislation allowing the military to help law enforcement officials, upgrading law enforcement equipment, withholding foreign aid from Third World countries involved in the export of drugs, and stiffening penalties for drug dealing. However, more and more experts in the field agree that what we need instead of more laws is creative thinking to come up with ways to counteract the demand for drugs rather than the supply. With every shipment of organic dope stopped at the border, fresh supplies of homemade synthetics find their way to the market.

8 The Synthetics: Rolling the Dice with Death

In 1972, Edward M. Brecher and the editors of the Consumer Union's Report in *Licit and Illicit Drugs* (Little, Brown) warned the public, the politicians, and law enforcement officials of the threat of concentrated drug forms and emphasized the danger of contaminated synthetic drugs spreading on the black market.

That was fourteen years ago. The documented historical study, which should have been made required reading by all policy makers, accurately forecasted the effects of this country's drug policies on black-market trends:

> What prohibition does accomplish is to raise prices and thus to attract more entrepreneurs to the black market . . . What prohibition also achieves is to convert the market from relatively bland, bulky substances to more hazardous concentrates which are more readily smugglable and marketable—from opium smoking to heroin mainlining, from coca leaves to cocaine, from marijuana to hashish. Again, prohibition opens the door to adulterated and contaminated drugs—methyl alcohol, "ginger jake," pseudo-LSD, adulterated heroin.

The trend continues today as cocaine is converted to Crack and heroin is replaced with synthetic heroin that has crippled and killed hundreds of users.

Sales of illegal narcotics and cocaine currently exceed $100 billion annually. In the past five years cocaine deaths have tripled. Heroin has become an acceptable if not a chic drug to smoke or skin-pop. Law enforcement is arresting more dealers and distributors selling both cocaine and heroin as drugs to be used in a variety of combinations. As more users experiment with the traditional narcotics and cocaine, the risk of sampling a deadly synthetic dramatically increases.

Americans appear to be as uninformed about the predictable effects of the organic drugs as they are about the synthetics. Coroners' reports and National Institute on Drug Abuse statistics have been warning users for more than a decade. Yet warnings and statistics couldn't accomplish what the deaths of Len Bias and Don Rodgers accomplished in a single instant. Their deaths announced to millions of shocked Americans that cocaine kills. Lots of other not-so-famous "recreational users" died, but their deaths didn't make headlines. Maybe they should have. But would anyone have listened?

One week after Maryland basketball star Len Bias died from a cocaine overdose, a freebaser confided that his dealer had just returned with $16,000 in cash after selling cocaine to the bat boy of a major league baseball team. The bat boy acted as distributor to the players. The dealer said Bias's death hadn't affected his sales, but had made him nervous. The possibility of another big-leaguer dying and all the publicity and cops and investigations and, well, it just made him nervous. Maybe he wouldn't sell to them anymore.

And yet when someone dies from food or drug tampering at a supermarket, the entire country is thrown into a panic and grocery shelves in state after state are emptied. We have hundreds of users dead from tainted synthetic heroin; we have an epidemic of Parkinson's disease on the West Coast, but neither tragedy has any effect on black-market sales. Why?

Part of the problem stems from an ignorance of the black market and how it works. The notion that we are dealing with some nebulous Darth Vader-like organization confined to the bowels of Harlem is a myth dispelled when we listen to clandestine chemists, dealers, and drug runners talk about their trade.

They confirm what law enforcement experts have been telling us for years: that the black market is the epitome of free enterprise, consisting of thousands of private businesses—financiers, manufacturers, chemists, drug runners, chemical wholesalers, distributors, dealers, subdealers, dealer-users, the fellow next door, all of whom operate for profit within a framework of tough competition.

They describe the synthetic narcotic business as a lucrative enterprise attracting more and more amateur and professional chemists experienced in the manufacture of other synthetics like PCP and speed. They tell you the synthetics are cheap to cook up, easy to disguise and sell, and tough for law enforcement to detect. They tell you the synthetic drug trade is here to stay for no other reason than it's a great way to make money. Hearing it from the source is believing it.

The black-market chemist arrested for manufacturing fentanyl analogs linked to deaths on the West Coast will go to trial for breaking FDA regulations. That he will never again be on the street cooking up dope is unlikely.

A second chemist arrested for the manufacture of synthetic heroin will plead guilty to manufacturing methamphetamine instead.

A third chemist arrested for sales of synthetic heroin on the East Coast is awaiting sentencing.

A fourth chemist serving time for the manufacture of PCP and linked to the Parkinson's disease epidemic from previously manufactured synthetic narcotics has exhibited symptoms of the disease while in prison. Meanwhile, a special task force is investigating his former associates thought to be manufacturing synthetic narcotics somewhere on the West Coast.

Bootleg recipes for the synthetic narcotics are for sale on both coasts. As of this writing, investigations of synthetic narcotics are underway in Florida, Delaware, Michigan, California, Louisiana, New York, New Jersey, and Texas. For every lab taken down, three more go undetected.

A crucial recommendation made by the Consumer Union's report fourteen years ago, one that continues to go unheeded today, is that we stop wasting money and energy on unreachable goals like wiping out drug supplies and concentrate our energy instead on discouraging nonusers from experimenting with drugs.

Altering the demand for drugs is the real source and solution to this problem. Demand diminishes when a product is known to be lethal rather than merely dangerous. Synthetic narcotics have randomly killed and crippled. Purchasing narcotics off the street that may be synthetic—which the buyer has no way of knowing—has become a high stakes gamble. The user gambles his life.

This book is a small attempt to get that message across and, in so doing, set a new direction for drug education.

Users and nonusers alike need to be informed about the devastating effects of heroin, cocaine, and their synthetic impersonators. A visit to a big city hospital where young adults might observe a baby suffering narcotic withdrawal is an unforgettable lesson in the pharmacological and toxicological effects of narcotics. The chance to see a three-year-old still unable to walk or talk because of the lingering dissociative effects of PCP will say more than a dozen texts on the subject. To meet the victims of synthetic drug poisoning—themselves once healthy young adults—and to witness first-hand the horribly disfiguring symptoms of Parkinson's disease and Huntington's Chorea is to see a powerful demonstration of what these drugs do.

A visit to the coroner's office can be instructive. The toxicologist can give a rundown on the past year's drug casualties. A local physician might spare the time to describe in vivid detail what those last few moments of life are like before convulsions and death from a drug overdose.

For parents to believe that it is the government's responsibility to keep kids off drugs is to turn their backs on their children. Learning to treasure our health and a certain quality of life begins in the home.

Sending six Black Hawk army helicopters and 150 military personnel into the Bolivian mountains hoping to get Crack off our streets may be well intentioned, but it is also naive. No matter how reassuring it is to blame Congress, and local, state, and federal law enforcement—or parents, for that matter—the bottom line is that individuals must be made responsible for themselves.

We have members of the medical profession and the media, senators and representatives, researchers and law enforcement officials who will agree that serious changes must be made in the way this country is trying to solve its drug problems. The time is right for those individuals to take the courageous step forward and suggest the unconventional. We must give them our support.

In the final analysis, designer drugs have become the very best reason not to do drugs. After all, what has life got to offer besides a twenty-minute artificial high? Plenty.

Glossary

addiction—compulsive physiological and psychological need for habit-forming drugs, such as caffeine, alcohol, nicotine, cocaine, and heroin.

adulterate—to make impure by the addition of a foreign or inferior substance; to prepare for sale by replacing more valuable substance with inert ingredients.

alkaloid—any of numerous usually colorless, complex and bitter organic bases (as morphine or codeine) containing nitrogen and usually oxygen that occur especially in seed plants.

alpha-methyl fentanyl—the first illicit fentanyl analog to be identified on the street.

ammonium hydroxide—a) the basic compound which results when ammonia gas reacts with water; b) the active ingredient in household ammonia cleaner. When ammonium hydroxide is added to a water solution of cocaine hydrochloride, the cocaine (base) is freed from the HCl molecule.

amphetamine—a white crystalline compound used as a central nervous system stimulant that raises energy levels, reduces appetite and the need for sleep and produces euphoria. Chronic use rapidly produces tolerance resulting in escalating doses. Amphetamine and its derivatives are sometimes misrepresented as cocaine on the street.

analgesia—insensibility to pain without loss of consciousness.

analog—a) a chemical compound structurally similar to another but differing often by a single element of the same valence and group of the periodic table as the element it replaces; b) a chemical substance that exhibits a minor modification of the root drug form, often exhibiting a marked increase in the effect of the drug.

anesthesia—loss of sensation with or without loss of consciousness.

base smoking—the heating of cocaine base using a glass pipe to vaporize it in order to inhale the vapors.

balloon—used as package for the sale of heroin.

black market—illicit trade of goods in violation of official regulations; the street or location where trade takes place.

bromocriptine—a fast-working drug used as temporary treatment for cocaine withdrawal by blocking the euphoric effects of cocaine and the user's craving for cocaine; in high doses it can produce side effects including dizziness and blackouts.

byproduct—a secondary unexpected substance produced in addition to the intended principal product.

caffeine—an alkaloid which is a stimulant and found in coffee, tea, and numerous other plants.

cardiopulmonary—involving the heart and the lungs.

cardiorespiratory—involving the heart and respiratory system.

cardiovascular—involving the heart and blood vessels.

C.D.C.—Centers for Disease Control.

China White—pure Southeast Asian heroin; name used to refer to synthetic designer heroins sold to unsuspecting users as real heroin and subsequently linked to several overdose deaths.

C.N.O.A.—California Narcotics Officers Association.

coca—a shrub originating in the Andes from which the alkaloid cocaine is derived.

cocaine—a bitter crystalline alkaloid that is obtained from coca leaves and is used as a local anesthetic and a stimulant of the central nervous system.

cocaine hydrochloride—a salt form of pure cocaine which has an electrical charge and is soluble in water.

cop—(to cop) slang for the purchase of heroin.

Council of Cooks—alleged group of clandestine chemists, hoping to stop others like themselves thought to be responsible for the deaths and disease linked to contaminated and extremely potent synthetic drugs.

Crack—marketing name for cocaine that has been freebased by street dealers, using soda bicarbonate, and sold as small pellets in vials at affordable prices.

Crystal—slang for methamphetamine.

cut—a substance used to dilute an active ingredient.

D.E.A.—Drug Enforcement Administration.

designer drugs—a) term christened by Dr. Gary Henderson of U.C. Davis to refer to state of the art chemistry on the black market; b) new, untested, legal synthetic drugs mimicking the effects of illicit narcotics, hallucinogens, stimulants, and depressants; c) concentrated or varied forms of existing illicit drugs renamed and marketed for certain income groups.

detox—to remove the effects of a drug from the body.

dopamine—a neurotransmitter responsible for what individuals experience as euphoria and pleasure among other things; stimulates an area of the brain affecting voluntary movement.

Dust—slang for phencyclidine (PCP).

ether (diethyl)—the solvent traditionally used to make cocaine hydrochloride; it is extremely flammable and forms explosive peroxides on exposure to air.

Ecstasy—marketing name given to MDMA—a combination stimulant and hallucinogen related to methamphetamine and MDA; currently illegal.

euphoria—a sense of well-being and exhilaration.

fentanyl—generic name for synthetic narcotic; trade name is Sublimaze, used as painkiller in surgery.

forensic labs—police labs.

freebase—the slang term for the alkaline form of the cocaine molecule which is used for smoking.

gas chromatography—an analytic technique which separates a mixture of compounds from each other in a stream of moving gas which passes through a specially designed tube.

heat—law enforcement.

hepatitis—inflammation of the liver.

heroin—a physiologically addictive narcotic made from morphine and more potent than morphine. Sold on the black market in powder form ranging in color from white to dark brown and sold also as black tar, having a bitter taste and smelling like vinegar.

holding—to be in possession of heroin, to be carrying heroin bodily.

Huntington's Chorea—a chronic nervous disorder marked by spastic muscle movements.

hype—user who shoots heroin.

inosital—a type of sugar-alcohol which is frequently used to adulterate cocaine hydrochloride.

intermediate—the form a drug takes in a two-step (or more) procedure before final synthesis is complete.

intravenous—(I.V.), using a drug by injecting it into a vein.

junk—heroin.

Let's Keep Drugs Clean—motto of Council of Cooks (black-market organization opposed to "designer chemists" killing and crippling users).

lactose—a sugar also known as milk-sugar which is sometimes used to adulterate cocaine hydrochloride.

lidocaine—a local anesthetic frequently used to adulterate cocaine hydrochloride or sold as cocaine hydrochloride itself.

mannitol—a) a sugar-alcohol commonly used to adulterate cocaine; b) mild laxative.

mass spectrometer—an instrument which fragments and separates molecules into various building blocks which can frequently provide enough information to reconstruct what the original molecule looked like.

meperidine—trade name Demerol; a synthetic analgesic (painkiller) developed as a morphine substitute. It is the narcotic most often abused by health professionals.

methadone—a synthetic addictive narcotic drug used for the relief of pain and used as a substitute narcotic for heroin.

methamphetamine—a synthetic central nervous system stimulant referred to as "speed," "Crystal," or "Crank" on the black market.

methyl benzoate—a compound with a strong wintergreen aroma. It is produced when an extreme amount of hydrochloric acid is added to crude cocaine to produce salt cocaine, resulting in some decomposition of the cocaine molecule. It is formed from the decomposition products and is sometimes sold on the street as cocaine itself.

morphine—a bitter crystalline addictive narcotic base which makes up between 4% and 21% of the raw opium. On the black market it might look like white crystals. For medical use it is prepared as tablets or injectable solutions. It has no odor and darkens with age. It is most commonly converted to codeine, a prescription opioid.

nanogram—one-billionth of a gram.

narcotic—a drug that in moderate doses dulls the senses, relieves pain, and induces profound sleep, but in excessive doses causes stupor, coma, or convulsions.

N.I.D.A.—National Institute on Drug Abuse.

N.I.M.H.—National Institute of Mental Health.

neurodegenerative—a deterioration of the nervous system.

neurotransmitter—signal-carrying chemicals that broadcast messages within the body's network of nerves.

norepinephrine—neurotransmitter responsible for an individual's alertness, energy, and assertiveness.

nystagmus—a rapid, involuntary oscillation of the eyeballs.

opium—a bitter, brownish, addictive narcotic drug that consists of the dried juice of the opium poppy. It is harvested from poppies grown in the Middle East, the Far East, Mexico and more recently in the United States.

parafluoro fentanyl—illicit fentanyl analog (designer heroin).

Parkinson's disease—a progressive nervous disease characterized by tremor and weakness of resting muscles and a peculiar gait.

pharmacological effects—physiological reactions to drugs.

phenylpropanolamine—a compound used in antihistamines and non-prescription diet pills, similar to amphetamines in chemistry and sometimes used to adulterate cocaine.

pinned—intoxicated.

precursor—a substance from which another substance is formed.

procaine—both a local and spinal anesthetic; sometimes used to adulterate cocaine.

psychoactive—affecting the mind or behavior.

psilocybin—a hallucinogenic organic compound obtained from a fungus (mushroom).

pulmonary edema—excess accumulation of fluid in the lungs.

PWA—Person With AIDS.

reagent—a substance used in a chemical reaction to produce other substances. It usually does not become part of the finished substance.

rock cocaine—a) a form of cocaine hydrochloride which is dense, unlayered, and similar in appearance to rock salt; b) freebased cocaine using the soda bicarbonate method and sold from "rock houses" on the West Coast.

run—(to be on a run), to be using chronically.

sens—high grade marijuana.

serotonin—neurotransmitter responsible for the regulation of sleep and appetite.

snorting—taking a drug by inhalation through the nose.

solvent—a liquid used to dissolve materials, or to aid in separation or transfer of other substances. It does not become part of the finished product.

step on—to dilute by adding adulterants in order to increase quantity to be sold and thereby earn more profits.

tetracaine—a local anesthetic sometimes used to adulterate cocaine.

THC—active ingredient in marijuana.

3-methyl fentanyl—illicit fentanyl analog (designer heroin) linked to overdose deaths.

toxicological—effects and properties of poisons.

toxin—a poisonous substance of animal or vegetable origin, especially one produced by micro-organisms.

tweaked—extreme nervous agitation resulting from methamphetamine intoxication.

Bibliography

Blaustein, Mordecai P., Dieter K. Bartschat and Roger G. Sorensen. *Proceedings of the National Academy of Sciences,* January 1986.

Brecher, Edward M. *Licit and Illicit Drugs.* Boston: Little, Brown, 1972.

Burroughs, William S. *Junky.* Baltimore: Penguin Books, 1953.

Cohen, Sidney. "Psychotherapy with LSD: Pro and Con." Presented at the LSD Conference: *The Use of LSD.* 1965.

Dackis, Charles A., and Mark S. Gold. "New Concepts in Cocaine Addiction: The Dopamine Depletion Hypothesis." *Neuroscience and Biobehavioral Reviews* 9 (1985).

Drug Enforcement Administration. "Schedules of Controlled Substances." *Federal Register* 50 (29 October 1985).

"Effects of PCP, Cocaine on Unborn: A Tragic Picture." *Los Angeles Times,* 5 December 1985.

Emboden, William. *Narcotic Plants.* New York: Macmillan, 1979.

Gold, Mark S. *800-Cocaine.* New York: Bantam Books, 1984.

Griffith, H. Winters. *Prescription and Non-Prescription Drugs.* Tuscon: HP Books, 1983.

Hales, Robert E., and Allen J. Frances. *American Psychiatric Association Annual Review.* Vol. 4. Washington, D.C.: American Psychiatric Press, 1985.

Henderson, Gary L. "The Pharmacology and Toxicology of the Fentanyls (China White)." Dept. of Pharmacology, School of Medicine, U.C., Davis.

"Huntington's Chorea: choreiform symptoms experienced by methamphetamine abusers." Prepared by the Divisional Intelligence Unit, San Francisco Field Division, July 1986.

Kline, David. "The Anatomy of Addiction." *Equinox* 4 (September-October 1985).

Kozel, Nicholas, and Edgar Adams. *Cocaine Use in America: Epidemiologic and Clinical Perspectives.* Monograph 61. Washington, D.C.: National Institute on Drug Abuse, 1985.

Lamar, Jacob V., Jr. "Crack." *Time,* 2 June 1986.

Langston, William J. *The Dangers of the Designer Drug Phenomenon.* Reported and prepared for the Senate Budget Committee Hearing, 18 July 1985.

Latimer, Dean. "MPTP: 'Brain Damage Dope' Floods West Coast Suburbs." *High Times,* October 1985.

Lee, David. *Cocaine Handbook: An Essential Reference.* Berkeley: And/Or Press, 1981.

Lewin, Roger. "Parkinson's Disease: An Environmental Cause?" *Agricultural Science,* 19 July 1985.

Linder, Ronald L., Steven Lerner, and Stanley Burns. *PCP: The Devil's Dust.* Belmont, Calif.: Wadsworth Publishing, 1981.

Luby, E. D., B. D. Cohen, G. Rosenbaum, J. J. Gottlieb, and R. Kelly. "Study of a New Schizophrenic Drug—Sernyl." *AMA Arch Neuro Psychiatry* (1959).

Luisada, P. V. *The Phencyclidine Psychosis: Phenomenology and Treatment.* Monograph 21. Washington, D.C.: National Institute on Drug Abuse, 1978.

Maranto, Gina. "Coke: The Random Killer." *Discover,* March 1985.

Markev, S. P., N. Castagnoli, Jr., A. J. Trevor, and J. J. Kopin. *MPTP—A Neurotoxin Producing A Parkinsonian Syndrome.* Orlando, Fla.: Academic Press, 1985.

Morganthaul, Tom, Mark Miller, Janet Hack, and Jeannie DeQuinne. "Kids and Cocaine." *Newsweek,* 17 March 1986.

Mothner, Ira, and Alan Weitz. *How to Get Off Drugs.* New York: Rolling Stone Press, 1985.

Petersen, Robert C., and Richard C. Stillman. *Phencyclidine (PCP) Abuse.* Monograph 21. Washington, D.C.: National Institute on Drug Abuse, 1978.

Quirion, R. "Stereospecific Displacement of . . . (PCP) Receptor Binding by an Enantiomeric Pair of PCP Analogs." *European Journal Pharmacology* (1981).

Shafer, Jack. "Designer Drugs." *Science,* March 1985.

Spotts, James V., and Carol A. Spotts. *Use and Abuse of Amphetamine and Its Substitutes.* Washington, D.C.: National Institute on Drug Abuse, 1980.

Stafford, Peter. *Psychedelics Encyclopedia.* Berkeley: And/Or Press, 1977.

Stark, Richard Vance. *Drug Manufacturers' Bible.*

"Street-Drug Contaminant Causing Parkinsonism." *Morbidity and*

Mortality Weekly Report (Centers for Disease Control), 22 July 1984.

Taylor, Ronald A., Adam Weisman and Ted Gest. "Killer Drugs, New Facts, New Enemies." *U.S. News & World Report,* 28 July 1986.

Thomas, Evan. "The Enemy Within." *Time,* 15 September 1986.

Thompson, Hunter. *Fear and Loathing in Las Vegas.* New York: Warner Books, 1971.

U.S. Congress. Senate. Committee on the Budget. *Designer Drugs: Hearings.* 99th Cong., 18 July 1985.

U.S. Department of Justice. Drug Enforcement Administration. *Controlled Substances Analogs.* Washington, D.C., Government Printing Office, 1985.

Verebey, Karl, and Mark S. Gold. "Endorphins and Mental Disease." *Handbook of Neurochemistry* 19 (1985).

Vincent, J. P. et al. "Interaction of Phencyclidine with a Specific Receptor in Rat Brain Membranes." *Proceedings of the National Academy of Science: USA* (1979).

Zukin and Zukin. "Specific Phencyclidine Binding in Rat Central Nervous System." *Proceedings of the National Academy of Science: USA* (1979).

Index